Youth Workers, Stuckness, and the Myth of Supercompetence

Youth workers and other helping professionals regularly find themselves in situations where, despite their experience and education, they simply do not know what to do or how to respond to the circumstances facing them. This book takes up the moment of not-knowing as experienced by youth workers, providing accessible phenomenological descriptions of the experience as lived by several youth workers. In addition to exploring the five dominant themes of the experience, the book situates not-knowing in the larger context of the helping professions and the professionalization of youth work in the United States. It concludes with a discussion of the implications of not-knowing for individual youth workers, for improved practice through integrated clinical and professional supervision, and for the field as a whole.

This book will be helpful to practitioners and supervisors in youth work and other helping professions. Youth workers will be able to find themselves reflected in and readily engage with the narratives. Direct service workers and supervisors will benefit from the focuses on practical implications of not-knowing and opportunities for action to help resolve its negative outcomes. Finally, interpretive researchers and students will benefit from the step-by-step description of how to conduct phenomenological investigations.

This book was published as a special issue of *Child & Youth Services*.

Ben Anderson-Nathe is Assistant Professor in Child and Family Studies at Portland State University in Portland, Oregon, where he also coordinates undergraduate practicum experiences for students entering the fields of youth work, social work, and education. His areas of research and teaching are youth development, youth worker training and development, human sexuality, anti-oppression organizing and education, and the bridges between theory and practice in public policy, health, and social services.

Youth Workers, Stuckness, and the Myth of Supercompetence

Not knowing what to do

Ben Anderson-Nathe

Routledge
Taylor & Francis Group
LONDON AND NEW YORK

First published 2010 by Routledge
2 Park Square, Milton Park, Abingdon, Oxon, OX14 4RN

Simultaneously published in the USA and Canada
by Routledge
270 Madison Avenue, New York, NY 10016

Routledge is an imprint of the Taylor & Francis Group, an informa business

Typeset in Times by Value Chain, India

British Library Cataloguing in Publication Data
A catalogue record for this book is available from the British Library

ISBN10: 0-415-99772-0 (h/b)
ISBN10: 0-415-99773-9 (p/b)

ISBN13: 978-0-415-99772-0 (h/b)
ISBN13: 978-0-415-99773-7 (p/b)

CONTENTS

Chapter 1

My Stomach Fell Through the Floor: The Moment of Not-Knowing What to Do

SUMMARY. Youth workers routinely experience moments in their professional practice with young people when, despite their experience and training, they are simply at a loss for what to do, how to respond, and how to be helpful to the youth. These experiences of not-knowing are seldom shared with other youth workers, which contributes to a climate of shame and humiliation. Professional supervision seldom attends to how youth workers experience these moments and their personal and vocational costs. This study presents a phenomenological investigation of how youth workers experience moments of not knowing what to do, identifies five central themes of the experience, and makes recommendations for improved youth work practice and supervision. This chapter presents the research question and its significance to the field of American youth work.

WHERE IT BEGAN

On an overnight shift a couple of months into my career, I was the sole adult in the basement sleeping area of the house. Every 15 minutes, I conducted bed checks according to house policy to ensure that all the residents were safe and accounted for. The procedure included walking from room to room, standing in the doorway, and shining a small flashlight on each bed, not to wake the sleeper but just to account for each young person.

At the end of one of these checks, I stood in the doorway of a girls' room and aimed the flashlight at the first three of four beds inside. When the beam hit the last bed, the girl sat up halfway as if awake, took several deep, gasping breaths, and started waving her arms in front of her body, screaming, "No, no, no! Get away! Get *away!*" Her screams continued, and her entire body started shaking. "No! No! Get away! Get *off me!*" She had probably heard me walking up and down the hall and partially woke up, looking toward the door. There she saw the shape of an adult man holding a light and blocking her doorway, the hallway light behind him obscuring any identifying features. In her half-awake, half-asleep daze, my figure blended in with that of the rapist whose recent assault brought her into our care.

I stood in the doorway, paralyzed and sweating, deafened by her screams and the blood pounding in my ears, wishing I knew what to do. I wanted to cry, but I also wanted to console. I wanted to hide, but I also wanted to reassure the other youth that everything would be okay. As youth in the house began to wake up, and as my shift partner appeared from the staircase to investigate, my body betrayed me and I shook. I had done everything according to my training, according to procedure, and still I had triggered an emotional crisis for a young woman whose safety I was supposed to guarantee. I was completely lost; I had no idea how to react to a situation I was sure I should have been prepared to handle. All my education, experience, training, and knowledge left me totally unprepared to respond to the situation; I could only stare as my stomach fell through the floor.

Backing away from the door into the area near the staff desk, my mind was racing and I felt dizzy and disoriented. First came the practical questions: What did I do wrong? What should I have done differently? How could I have allowed this to happen? What could I have done to make the situation better? Then the existential ones: What kind of youth worker was I?! Not only could I not prevent this trauma, I actually caused this incident! Did this mean that I was just not cut out for this work? What if I was fundamentally unworthy of this position? And then the personal: What would other people think about me—other residents, my colleagues, my supervisors? What did it mean about me that this has happened?

The experience awoke in me the sudden and troubling realization that as a youth worker, I will continue to find myself in situations where I do not know what to do. This realization, combined with the understanding that in many such situations other people will look to me expecting a professional and competent response and find none, shook my newly emerging youth work identity. What did it mean to enter this field, to remain in it, to think of and present myself as a youth worker if I lack the competence to respond effectively?

I met with my supervisor the next day, after the incident reports had been written, the kids had been talked to, and the other staff had all been debriefed. The content of our meeting was intended to reassure me, I know: I had done nothing wrong. There was nothing I could have done to anticipate the flashback. In residential treatment, and particularly in crisis residential centers, these things happen. Youth enter the program from any number of backgrounds and with a wide range of often traumatic experiences and issues. Sometimes, the effects of these experiences leak out at unexpected times. Although difficult for the young woman and possibly the other youth in the house, what had happened was certainly not the result of my wrongdoing. In fact, the incident probably provided a helpful vignette for this young woman's process of reflection and healing. With these assurances from my supervisor, our meeting satisfied the practical questions of the night before.

It did not, however, satisfy my existential and personal or professional doubt. I left my shift a few hours after my supervision, still feeling at a loss to understand or be able to talk about what had happened the night before. I felt resolved about the technical details. I knew I would not be reprimanded. I was convinced that the situation could not have been prevented. Nonetheless, what had happened haunted me, and no one—not my supervisor or my fellow residential counselors—asked me what the experience had been like for me. For weeks, I continued to second-guess myself in silent isolation, to wonder about my ability (or in a strange way, my *right*) to do youth work. Was it even ethical for me to continue? I found little opportunity to explore these questions. It was hard for me to know whether others had ever shared this experience; I knew my colleagues simply must have, but their stories never reached me. Privately, I feared that what I rationally knew (others experience this, too) might actually not be true. The question lingered with me: What if my peers are simply better at their jobs than I am at mine? The anxiety of this possibility—what I have come to call the *myth of* supercompetence—and its implications kept me silent. Weeks went by, and the experience faded from the everyday to one remembered day.

NOT-KNOWING IN CONTEXT

Months later, I found myself in another situation of the same not-knowing-what-to-do, and I again cycled through a series of very similar questions. The events of the two scenarios were wholly different, but my experience of them was the same. Many years down the road, I can tell story after story of these experiences. I hear them in my research, my teaching, and in workshops and community conversations with other youth workers.[1] I now know that my colleagues shared these experiences. The details of the events differ, certainly, but the tone of the experience remains consistent. Also consistent is the tendency on the part of youth workers and supervisors alike to structure supervision in such a way that it analyzes the technical and practical questions but leaves our deeper existential and personal reactions unexamined. Put differently, much of our supervision, particularly around moments of not-knowing, focuses almost entirely on addressing practical concerns, often at the expense of the emotional, vocational, and personal dimensions of these experiences and of our work.

In a recent workshop on the experience of not-knowing among clinical social workers, a participant took issue with my statements about the state of supervision in the helping professions. Supervisors, he argued, are trained to help their staff address these deeper personal and existential questions while also responding to the practical needs a situation may present. I did not doubt the truth of his statement then, and I do not doubt it now. Having heard dozens of youth workers and other helping professionals disclose and describe their experiences of not-knowing, however, I am more convinced than ever that even as supervisors believe they create space for their staff to process these experiences, their staff often perceive the supervision differently. Despite the skill and supportive intentions of their supervisors, many youth workers describe a climate of silence around the personal and professional toll exacted by these experiences of not-knowing. In order for youth workers to sustain themselves in their work, and for the field to sustain itself, this climate must change.

Exposing how youth workers experience themselves in situations of not knowing how to respond, not knowing enough about a situation, or not knowing what to do helps change the climate of youth work practice. These episodes of uncertainty, confusion, and doubt are the moments that may best define the as-yet amorphous field of youth work: unexpected encounters with people and situations emerge and crises are commonplace. Youth work practitioners are often in situations of doubt and uncertainty, finding themselves in conditions like that described above for which their training, education, and experience—however vast—leave them entirely unprepared.

These are moments that might, at any other time, present no dilemma whatsoever. One hallmark of the experience of not-knowing is that it cannot entirely be explained or anticipated. Situations a youth worker manages instinctively and flawlessly on Monday may get that same worker completely stuck in not-knowing on Thursday. For this reason, we cannot speak merely of specific instances likely to engender the phenomenon. We cannot attribute not-knowing to inexperience or faulty practice. And we must be careful how we frame and discuss the experience itself. Many terms come close to naming the phenomenon (including existential incapacity, helplessness, doubt, futility, and more), but none has captured the experience or struck a chord among youth workers like not-knowing or being stuck. These terms have consistently resonated in conversations with other youth workers, evoking an immediate "aha!" and, invariably, the telling of a story. The stories I have heard are often shared in ways similar to how one might talk about a war wound or a challenge overcome; they either earn bragging rights for the survivor or function as comic relief. Sharing the details of the events, however, which is how these stories are most often told, is not enough. As my own experience of the rape flashback suggests, we must explore the human cost of these experiences, as well.

We most often focus our supervisions and conversations with colleagues on answering technical questions related to the situation, exploring our experience in a professional, practical context. In more focused moments, we occasionally probe the experience for its meanings along the lines of what that professional experience means for the practice of our vocation and careers. While these discussions are helpful in providing context for and insight into preventing those same situations from occurring again in those same ways, they do little to provide space for authentic reflection on our practice and ourselves as practitioners.

Parker Palmer (1998) has written about this reflection among teachers and other educators. He has called for increased attention to the benefits of professional reflection, and his recommendations for increased attention to the inner landscape of educators' lives also apply to youth workers. But even in professional reflection, we seldom attend to the experience of not-knowing from the perspective of youth worker as both professional *and* human being. Generally, we fail to look for the meaning made of the experience of *self* in moments of not-knowing. Developing familiarity with and facility talking about our stories of not-knowing from the perspective of the whole self allows youth workers to connect the lived and reflected experiences of the phenomenon.

Absent an understanding of the meanings ascribed to these moments, and specifically to themselves as experiencers *of* these moments, I fear that youth workers will continue to muddle through the cycles of self-doubt and existential or vocational angst that accompany them. Muddling through might not be a fundamentally bad thing; even in muddling, we make meaning. However, without deliberate reflection and integration of this meaning into the context of past and future experiences (calling conscious attention to the muddling of yesterday and how it relates to the muddling of today and tomorrow), the potential utility of the experience diminishes (Dewey, 1938). Through phenomenological inquiry and reflection, we can clarify youth workers' experiences of self in these moments of not-knowing, providing greater depth to the experience and how youth workers and supervisors use these understandings to improve practice.

Of course, this experience of "stuckness," and the associated vocational and personal questions it brings, is not unique to youth workers. It is possible (perhaps even likely) that all professionals, surely all human services professionals, experience similar moments of not-knowing. The classroom is certainly a site for such experiences among teachers at all levels; disciplinary issues and particularly challenging or incendiary questions might well give rise to these moments. Law enforcement professionals likely experience something very similar, as well. Consequently, I am often asked why my work focuses principally on youth workers. The answer is simple: I have chosen to focus on youth workers because it is the ground from which I speak. It is my vocation and professional home, and it is the audience I have chosen to address, both in the United States and abroad. Still, focusing solely on youth work would present a limited and naïve exploration of not-knowing. Therefore, in chapter 2, I draw from other professions and disciplines to help situate the experience inside its larger context, with the hope that my presentation of how youth workers experience not-knowing might, in turn, act as a springboard for further study of the phenomenon in other professions.

Clarifying the audience, however, is not enough. I must also clarify my question and point to the tools with which it will be addressed. In the following chapters, I seek to understand something that is at once an abstraction and an often painful reality. The phenomenon of not-knowing is the abstraction; the experiencing of it is the reality. The distinction is important: it is one thing to attempt an understanding of a phenomenon but quite another to understand how people experience the situations where that phenomenon is revealed. Chapter 3 takes up this discussion, clarifying the tools used in exploring and understanding the phenomenon of not-knowing and, hopefully, providing a clear methodological map to help youth workers and others take up questions of experience and meaning remaining to be answered in other sectors of the helping professions. Gadamer (1989, as cited in Cohen, Kahn, & Steeves, 2000) wrote specifically of phenomenological inquiry in this case, emphasizing that hermeneutic phenomenology involves exploring how people understand (or experience) the world around them. Cohen et al. suggested that a Gadamerian approach to phenomenology focuses primarily on the experiencer's description and interpretation of a phenomenon rather than on the structure of the phenomenon itself (which is more of a Husserlian take on phenomenology). This line of inquiry reflects a balance of phenomenology and existential philosophy: phenomenology provides a means of openness to the experience, and existential philosophy frames that experience in terms of the meanings assigned to it by the experiencer. The emphasis is simultaneously on the phenomenon (not-knowing) and on the experience of that phenomenon for the experiencer (for instance, the questions, reactions, and effects that accompany situations of not-knowing).

Although the details of the events in which not-knowing discloses itself (Heidegger, 1962) vary widely, the phenomenon of not-knowing and its accompanying embodied responses (doubt and fear among them) is common. By probing youth workers' stories of not-knowing, attentive for what Parse (1987, p. 177) refers to as "the remembered, the now, and the not yet" about how they experience these moments and what meaning can be drawn from them, chapters 5 through 9 present discussions of youth workers' actual experiences and descriptions of not-knowing, including not only their physical reactions to the events but also the meanings they made of their stuckness after the fact.

Chapter 10 carries these descriptions of phenomenology and the experience of not-knowing into practical application, making its own contribution to the ongoing development of our field. Because most American youth workers identify themselves primarily as practitioners (and only secondarily, if at all, as theorists), the primary goal of my work is related to bettering our practice. In their study of nurses' desires to help others, Mitchell and Heidt (1994) suggested that phenomenological inquiry can contribute to a field's existing literature and practice by "enhancing understanding about human experience" (p. 119). Based on the stories they/we tell, not-knowing is a feature of youth workers' human experience, begging for increased understanding. This enhanced sense of the human condition is a valuable contribution in itself. But even more significantly, we must also be attentive to how understanding the experience can inform practice. This is certainly true of an investigation into the experience of self in situations of not-knowing. Understanding this experience can affect how youth workers respond in and after these situations, contributing to decreased burnout, increased professional/vocational competence, and improved training for supervisors and youth workers in direct practice. In this way, exploring the existential and vocational questions associated with moments of not-knowing may well influence the efficacy with which youth workers attend to the practical and technical questions in similar future moments.

Most significantly, however, my goal is simply to reach youth workers, to normalize the experience of not-knowing, to provide a language we can use to talk about ourselves in the context of this phenomenon, and to invite conversation—among colleagues and between youth workers and supervisors—about a feature of our work we all share but fear naming. I am encouraged by the courage of those youth workers whose voices appear in the following pages, those I have the honor and privilege of teaching, and those I meet in the community. Debunking the myth of supercompetence requires a culture shift in youth work practice, a shift that can only come through honest dialogue about our work. It is my hope that this book can help open that conversation.

NOTE

1. Youth work is here understood in the context of social pedagogy. Conceptualized in this way, American youth work draws from the traditions of interactive youth work, youth development, social education, and established (largely British and Canadian) models of professionalized youth work. Regardless of the sector of the field in which they practice, youth workers in this framework are those adults (a) who work primarily with youth (typically, people age 21 and younger), (b) whose work must include a learning and teaching component, and (c) with whom youth must enter voluntarily into the youth work relationship, direct the relationship in some significant way, and have the freedom to terminate the relationship (Jeffs & Smith, 1999; Krueger, 1998; Marsland, 1993; Milson, 1972).

REFERENCES

Cohen, M. Z., Kahn, D. L., & Steeves, R. H. (2000). *Hermeneutic phenomenological research: A practical guide for nurse researchers.* Thousand Oaks, CA: Sage.

Dewey, J. (1938). *Experience and education.* New York: MacMillan.

Gadamer, H. G. (1989). In J. Weinsheimer & D. G. Marshall, Trans. (Eds.) 2nd rev., *Truth and method.* New York: Crossroads.

Heidegger, M. (1962). In J. Macquarrie & E. Robinson, Trans. (Eds.), *Being and time.* New York: Harper & Row.

Jeffs, T., & Smith, M. (1999). The problem of "youth" for youth work. *Youth and Policy, 62*, 45–66.

Krueger, M. A. (1998). *Interactive youth work practice.* Washington, DC: CWLA.

Marsland, D. (1993). *Understanding youth: Issues and methods in social education.* St. Albans: Claridge.

Milson, F. (1972). *Why am I a youth worker? An examination of the goals and motives of youth workers.* London: National Association of Youth Clubs.

Mitchell, G. J., & Heidt, P. (1994). The lived experience of wanting to help another: Research with Parse's method. *Nursing Science Quarterly, 7*, 119–127.

Palmer, P. (1998). *The courage to teach: Exploring the inner landscape of a teacher's life.* San Francisco: Jossey-Bass.

Parse, R. R. (1987). *Nursing science: Major paradigms, theories, and critiques.* Philadelphia: Saunders.

Chapter 2

Contextualizing Not-Knowing: Terminology and the Role of Professional Identity

SUMMARY. This chapter provides a context for the concept of not-knowing, including a discussion of how the concept was framed. The experience of not-knowing in professional youth work is framed in relationship to other concepts explored by the social work and therapeutic literature (including vicarious trauma, helplessness, secondary trauma, and burnout), as well as those offered by the limited youth work and nursing literature discussing similar concepts (disruption and hurt, suffering, commitment in spite of conflict, and the struggle to go along when you do not believe). The standing of youth work in the professions and its own struggles to professionalize are explored, with attention to how not-knowing affects and is affected by these efforts.

In residential care, youth ministry, outdoor education, street outreach, and elsewhere, youth workers experience moments in their professional lives where they simply do not know how to respond. Often, these moments pass by without incident; they present merely a feature of the work and result in no long-standing crisis for the worker. Nevertheless, at other times the same events may be lived quite differently, bringing about panic and vocational questioning. These experiences often contribute to youth workers' professional anxiety, to the shame associated with a perception that they are unfit for their chosen career, and to burnout and its resulting departure from the field altogether.

Even in light of such consequences, however, the youth work literature has not sufficiently addressed how youth workers experience the moments of not-knowing. Despite the pervasiveness of not-knowing and how often youth workers find themselves stuck in such moments, neither the phenomenon itself, how youth workers live through it, nor what effects it has on their professional development and identity have been directly taken up in the youth work literature, either in the United States or abroad. For that matter, the absence of not-knowing from academic discourse is not limited to youth work; the research literature in related disciplines (education, social work, psychotherapy, and nursing among them) reflects a general reluctance to take up this phenomenon as well.

A ROSE BY ANY OTHER NAME: WHY "NOT-KNOWING"?

The absence of not-knowing in the literature may stem in part from the difficulty assigning a discrete name to the experience. While many youth workers and other helping professionals clearly encounter moments for which their experience and education leave them totally unprepared to respond, without a term to identify the experience and language to explore it, the phenomenon goes unnamed and ignored. Consequently, in conceptualizing this study, finding a suitable name for the experience presented one of the most significant challenges. Notions of existential anxiety, vocational doubt, and existential incapacity point toward the crisis youth workers often feel in response to the moment, but they fail to describe the actual experience itself. While naming not-knowing the "oh no!" experience or identifying it as helper helplessness captures the lived reaction to the moment, they too illustrate only a feature of the experience. They emphasize the in-the-moment reaction but fail to address its longer term impacts.

As a concept, "not-knowing" speaks to the experience as lived while also opening the possibility for larger implications; it addresses the core feature of the experience (the inability to conceptualize, understand, or respond to the moment) and foreshadows the implications (what if I never come back into knowing?). Further, not-knowing is itself a bounded term, defined by this study for the purposes of this specific study. While other terms might have applied, most of those considered have already been defined and used in other—albeit related—contexts. With the exception of Lesser's (2007) application of the term in the context of the psychotherapeutic relationship (where she uses not-knowing to describe therapists' willingness to allow themselves not to know and therefore remain open to their clients' exploration of issues or perceptions), not-knowing does not yet have the additional connotations of terminology used for related concepts.

NOT-KNOWING AND RELATED CONCEPTS

To the extent that not-knowing is taken into consideration in the social work, youth work, and associated literature, it emerges indirectly through concepts related to but still distinct from the experience as described in this study. These concepts tend to fall into four categories: those related to helplessness and the other; those related to the worker's response to the other; those describing the worker's experience; and those addressing the outcome of stress in the helping relationship. Each helps to contextualize a feature of not-knowing but none fully illustrates the experience.

Helplessness, Indecision, and the Other

Using Wittgenstein's (1953/2001) concept of family resemblance among words or concepts, one of the closest cousins of not-knowing is the notion of helper helplessness. After all, one of the hallmarks of the experience is the desire to be helpful and effective coupled with a profound and urgent sense of inability to do either. Workers experience feelings of impotence and an incapacity to formulate viable interventions or plans. Of course, these feelings of helplessness and indecision do not always result in the paralyzing experience of not-knowing. Nor are they limited to the helpers themselves; similar experiences of uncertainty and helplessness bring clients into the helping relationship in the first place. Social workers, youth workers, and therapists routinely work with clients who enter services exhibiting confusion and difficulty making sense of their environments. Teachers and crisis interventionists in schools regularly work with young people to unpack feelings of frustration and helplessness, identifying and testing out possible behavioral alternatives to resolve conflicts.

Hooker's (1976) discussion of learned helplessness in social work and therapeutic settings framed this confusion and indecision in the context of impaired functioning on the part of the client. Though related to not-knowing, this concept differs significantly from it, since it is presented as an issue solely for the client, not the worker. The issue is framed in terms of the development of a sense of impotence to change certain features of the individual's own life. Clients experience learned helplessness as the result of a retarded sense of self-efficacy, limited self-esteem, conditions of addiction, and the like. Despite recognizing the need for change, clients in these circumstances suffer a lack of internal resources necessary to bring about such change and become paralyzed (not entirely unlike youth workers in moments of not-knowing).

In this context, Hooker (1976) focused on equipping workers with the skills required to assess and empower their clients, thus resolving the sense of helplessness but not speaking to the worker's reaction to or possible identification with it. Likewise, the idea that helpers as well as the helped may well experience moments of helplessness and uncertainty is simply not considered. Nor does the literature consider the experience of helplessness itself, how people make meaning of their moments of helplessness, or come to redefine them. A few intervention methods, such as Life Space Crisis Intervention (LSCI), seek to explore where clients' helplessness or inability originated. Most such methods investigate the origin of helplessness with the goal of identifying alternative behaviors in order to respond to the conflict that helplessness has created. Even these methods focus solely on indecision or crisis as it relates to the client, not the worker (Long, Wood, & Fecser, 2001).

Not-Knowing in Response to the Other

In addition to considering the concepts of helplessness and whether these may refer equally to workers and clients, much can be learned from exploring those concepts linking not-knowing to the difficulty, trauma, pain, or uncertainty associated with responding to challenging material presented by clients. After all, the feelings of alienation, grief, and anxiety that often accompany moments of not-knowing share much in common with trauma reactions. Drawing from the psychotherapeutic and social work literature, these related issues include compassion fatigue (Figley, 2002; Garrett, 1999), secondary traumatic stress (Cornille & Meyers, 1999; Figley, 1995), and vicarious trauma (Bober & Regehr, 2006; Gabriel, 1994; McCann & Pearlman, 1990). All have much to offer a deep understanding of not-knowing in terms of what they convey about workers' short- and long-term reactions to traumatic events. Intrusive thoughts, survivor anxiety, and depression are common manifestations of secondary trauma that closely mirror the experiences of many youth workers following moments of not-knowing.

The utility of these terms is limited, however, by their reliance on a source of secondary trauma, experienced by the client and shared with the worker, as the origin of the worker's stress. That is, intrusive thoughts and depression result from the professional's experience witnessing the client's traumatic material, whether that comes from violence, abuse, war, or other sources. These concepts fail to address workers' traumatic responses to events that, in any other circumstance, would not have been traumatic, as is the case with many youth workers' moments of not-knowing. In many situations, after all, the events leading up to the moment of not-knowing are not, in themselves, particularly traumatic. Clearly related in some way to the effects of not-knowing on personal coping, professional identity, and existential doubt, these concepts nevertheless fail to capture the subtlety of the experience.

In his grounded theory of residential care programs for children and youth, Anglin (2002) takes up a similar thread, suggesting that correctly and sensitively interpreting and responding to young people's pain is one of the central challenges for residential youth workers. Nevertheless, even among seasoned workers, the strain of holding and addressing young people's pain can bring about a profound sense of anxiety, which Anglin refers to as "pain-based fear" (p. 112) within the workers themselves. This anxiety is difficult to manage and can create significant barriers between adults and youth in circumstances where workers are unable to effectively process and contain their own reactions. In moments of not-knowing, of course, such anxiety is exacerbated by workers' recognition of their own inability to respond.

Lived Experiences Related to Not-Knowing

Despite the absence of a complete description of not-knowing from the academic literature, there have nonetheless been a series of investigations into the lived experiences of related concepts. These differ from those notions described above in that they seek to describe how the concept is experienced and what meaning people make of it rather than its precursors and how it can be managed. This is particularly true in the nursing and existential psychology literature, with their careful attention to the lived experience of phenomena as they are encountered by nurses, other health care professionals, and patients.

Concerned with how people answer fundamental questions related to the meaning of experience, this literature has focused attention on the related issues of suffering (Shantall, 1998). The discourse surrounding suffering comes close to addressing not-knowing in some ways, suggesting that helpers experience a sense of suffering that is at once vicarious (secondarily experienced through their clients) and personal (the inability to alleviate suffering causes pain for helpers). As a central organizing principle for a study of not-knowing, however, this construct of suffering as experienced by helpers is insufficient. Clearly, in some circumstances, suffering may well be a feature of not-knowing. This, however, is not a foregone conclusion. Youth workers may find themselves in situations where they have no idea what to do but do not associate the experience with pain or punishment, as might be expected from suffering. Further, suffering may include a connotation of extended duration, as distinct from, say, merely pain. Not-knowing may be acute rather than chronic or may involve a number of episodes of varying duration and intensity.

Mitchell and Heidt (1994) examined the meaning of wanting to help in the context of nursing relationships with patients whose prognosis was questionable. This study offered insight into how nurses maintain hope in circumstances that seem dire and stressed the concept that living attentively within the constraints of a given situation can allow new possibilities to emerge. This insight offers much to the reflected experience of not-knowing, after the fact, when youth workers revisit the meaning they made of the experience. Kelley (1991) and Bournes (2000) have also contributed to related studies in nursing, focusing their attention on commitment in spite of conflict and the struggle to go along when you do not believe (in your work, its impact, its prognosis, etc.). The commitment to maintaining a relationship or a course of action, even in spite of uncertainty, doubt, or discomfort, may be common to many situations of not-knowing—the inability to withdraw from the situation despite discomfort in it—but it remains a tenuous connection.

In his exploration of residential child and youth care workers' occupational experiences, Arieli (1997) described pain and hurt as they featured in the work lives of staff. Framed as "disruptions" and "hurts," Arieli suggested that the former are moments in which the worker's work becomes more difficult, and the latter are those where the worker feels personally and emotionally hurt by the encounter. While disruptions remain a commonplace feature of residential work, hurts take a larger toll on the youth worker and can result in self-doubt and vocational questioning similar in many ways to that resulting from moments of not-knowing.

Further, Arieli (1997) found that that the degree of hurt (or, for this study, the negative associations of not-knowing) increases as the worker's investment in the youth or the situation increases—an observation that resonates with workers' descriptions of their reactions to not-knowing. Finally, Arieli's work suggested that residential workers seldom openly discuss their personal hurts, employing diverse strategies to manage the pain without having to personalize it and risk the recognition that they had been emotionally hurt.

Consequences of Not-Knowing

Discussions of not-knowing, vicarious trauma, pain-based fear among residential youth workers, and other related concepts often articulate a common consequence for failure to respond to these stressful experiences: burnout. When workers cannot effectively process, understand, share, and heal from the wounds they receive from these experiences, they often feel ineffective as helpers, alienated from and exhausted by their work, and frequently leave the field altogether (Shields, 1996).

The literature surrounding helper burnout, with its emphasis on the cumulative effects of uncertainty and unreflective practice, often emphasizes either personal characteristics of workers who tend to burn out and those who do not (McMullen & Krantz, 1988) or the job stressors (Lee & Ashforth, 1996) that contribute to it. Much of this work is based on the foundation laid by Maslach (1982), who identified an inventory of three dimensions contributing to burnout: emotional exhaustion, depersonalization, and diminished personal accomplishment. All personal characteristics, these factors maintain a focus on the individual rather than addressing the social, organizational, or cultural features that may also contribute to helping professionals' inability to sustain themselves in the field. There is more recent attention paid to social and environmental factors (Mattingly, 2006). This emerging literature holds some additional potential to situate not-knowing and its long-term effects.

In his cross-cultural study of child and youth care workers, Savicki (2002) broadened Maslach's work, exploring both the individual (personal) and cultural (environmental) precursors to and indicators of burnout. Savicki has suggested that burnout is the result of a series of interactions between personal and environmental factors within specific cultural contexts. A framework that offers much to an understanding of not-knowing and the stress or existential anxiety it may cause for youth workers, the interplay between personal and environmental influences, also sheds light on how some events—moments of not-knowing—may give rise to levels of personal and professional anxiety that foreshadow burnout for some workers, while the same events may generate a significantly less stressful reaction from others (or at other times).

While many discussions of burnout focus on the factors or variables giving rise to workers' inability to remain in the field, others emphasize strategies useful in diminishing burnout among helping professionals. In his discussion of managing compassion fatigue to prevent burnout, for instance, Figley (2002) has suggested that helpers must routinely seek support in their work and in managing the experienced trauma accompanying it from peers and other intimate relationships. The recommendation for enhanced supervision and peer support is indicative of a desire to minimize at least one of Maslach's (1982) contributors to burnout, emotional exhaustion, by developing an enriching and invigorating professional climate. However, in the case of youth workers' experiences of not-knowing, this is made particularly difficult because of the field's adherence to a standard of supercompetence and reluctance to admit to or share experiences to the contrary. This supercompetence, a core feature of not-knowing, will be explored in greater detail in subsequent chapters, as it may well represent one of the most significant contributors to alienation and burnout specific to youth work.

PROFESSIONALISM AND PROFESSIONAL IDENTITY

Given that moments of not-knowing occur in worker-client relationships and work settings and are informed by the expectations and roles inherent in a professional setting, it is essential to frame the discussion of these moments in terms of professionalism and professional identity among youth workers. Particularly in the United States, where youth work struggles to carve out a distinct niche in the helping professions, the theoretical foundations of professionalism and professional identity are central to a deep understanding of the meanings youth workers ascribe to their experiences of not-knowing.

Few training programs exist in the United States to train youth workers in a distinct professional or disciplinary perspective. Indeed, as Anglin (2002) observed among residential child and youth care workers, while most youth workers possess a college degree, only a fraction of those were trained in any of the helping professions or disciplines (including psychology or sociology). Most training and professional development occurs on the ground, as youth workers inform and model professional identity for one another. Lacking the formal training, licensure, and compensation or representation enjoyed by social workers and formal educators, for instance, youth work has developed a sense of itself as the helping professions' underdog—under fire from all sides, desperately trying to stake out its unique contribution to the field and the youth it serves but lacking the language to articulate its theoretical foundation and therefore clearly differentiate itself from the other professions.

Expanding on these criteria from a frame of reference emphasizing expertise and specialized knowledge, Schön's (1983) conceptualization of professional identity suggests that it rests in many ways upon the perceived ability of the professional to systematically and effectively respond to situations within his professional realm. In fact, the knowledge and ability with which the professional responds *define* the profession itself. Schein (1973) identified three characteristics essential to every profession (as distinct from fields that are nonprofessional): the presence of a unifying and underlying theory base, a scientific application of that theory, and the skills and attitudes required to implement the application. Within this construction, these characteristics elevate the professions and professionals above other forms of work and provide a certain privileged importance and competence to their practitioners.

Youth work's parent fields (education and social work) have long been accepted as professions, both clearly meeting Schein's (1973) criteria, as well as Kelly's (1990) assertion that acceptance as a profession requires the public's acceptance of that professional group's authority to act. Social work and education have met these standards; each has established standards of practice, theoretical foundations, and organizational structure. Both have struggled to develop, over the past century, the structure and appearance worthy of the professions, and, for the most part, these efforts are perceived to have been successful.

Youth work in the United States, on the other hand, possibly in response to its parents' achievements, continues to struggle with its professional identity and the public's acceptance of its unique contribution. Youth workers have long prided themselves on their atheoretical foundations, suggesting that an absence of canonical theory allows them a degree of openness with their clients and flexibility in drawing from effective interventions without regard to their disciplinary (or professional) ownership. On the other hand, as evidenced by current debates in British youth work regarding the introduction of a formalized youth work curriculum (Ord, 2004; Robertson, 2004; Stanton, 2004), others in the field have pushed for increased professionalization. Practitioners in child care and early childhood education have witnessed this tension in their own fields (Kelly, 1990; Powell, 1990), and it is an ongoing tension among American youth workers, as well.

Regardless to what degree the broader field of youth work has become professionalized (including the development of a body of theory, establishment of accepted best practices, and the creation of professional standards), many youth workers operate under a professional self-perception. That is, in accordance with Schein's definition, they see themselves as expected to possess a specialized body of knowledge—even if that knowledge remains practical, hands-on, local, and largely atheoretical—and the skills required to implement that knowledge. In spite of the absence of public affirmation of their authority, many youth workers hold themselves to a standard of practice at the level of social work and other helping professions; they expect themselves to be able to respond as would any other professional.

This self-expectation is complicated, to some degree, by the varied nature of the environments in which youth workers operate. It is difficult, with so little uniformity in practice, to foster the development of skills and aptitudes identified by Schein (1973) as crucial. Nonetheless, the ability to generalize one's practice from situation to situation is one hallmark of professional action. In his seminal piece on professional action, Schön (1983) identified that, in many cases, professionals are able to do just that: generalize competent and effective responses among varied circumstances. Suggesting that these responses result from a combination of knowledge-in-action and reflection-in-action, Schön (1983) highlighted the importance of improvisation in professional practice, as illustrated by examples from four professions.

The professional's ability to unite theory and specialized practice across unique circumstances is central to appreciating youth workers' experiences of not-knowing. Framing professionalism in terms of the worker's ability to encounter a scenario, assess its content, select the appropriate theoretical foundation for interpreting it, and then build a grounded response introduces tensions in the context of not-knowing. After all, appreciating the expectation of *knowing* what to do highlights the conflict created in one's professional identity when one finds oneself in a situation of *not*-knowing. In this way, the professional literature helps illustrate the conflict when youth workers find themselves in situations where their professional knowledge and skills leave them uncertain. Further, the need for public recognition of the emerging profession's authority to act underscores the stakes if youth workers admit they do not know; such admissions run the risk of undermining public perception and further denigrating youth work as a specialized profession in its own right.

Broadening Schein's (1973) conceptualization of the professions and exaggerating the conflicts facing youth workers in situations where they do not know, Brown (1980) added a moral component to her articulation of the professions' requisite features. She suggested that professions (and professionals) are distinct in that they "seek to perform some mission of service" (p. 18). That is, professionals bear an ethical responsibility for the delivery of their services. Physicians do not merely diagnose; they *treat*. Teachers do more than instruct; they *educate*. In both examples, the professional action carries an ethical obligation. Thus framed, the addition of an ethical component to the professional's identity is central to understanding the effects of not-knowing on a youth worker's experience of self.

In ways similar to nurses or physicians, youth workers often hold themselves ethically *responsible* for this professional conduct. In other words, seeing themselves as professionals, they accept the implied ethical charge to respond competently and effectively to any situation presented to them in the course of their work.[1] In so doing, youth workers place themselves in an untenable situation. If professional identity revolves around the ability to develop effective interventions based on specialized knowledge (which they are ethically obligated to do), what is the weight of the realization that one is unable to develop such an intervention? If youth workers cannot fulfill their ethical obligation to respond, what does that mean about their place in the profession? Although it does not provide answers to these questions, understanding the moral/ethical component of professional identity is useful in terms of developing a framework for youth workers' experiences of themselves in moments of not-knowing.

In religious and existential language (much of which has perfused, in recent years, other fields of care such as nursing), this is an issue of vocation. In this sense, vocation is understood less in its practical, work-related usage and more in terms of calling or purpose. Raatikainen (1997) has understood calling as a "deep internal desire to choose a task or profession which a person experiences as valuable and considers her own" (p. 1111). In other words, youth workers feel called to their profession precisely *because* of the moral element described by Brown (1989). They identify themselves with the profession, considering it central to them and themselves integral to it.

Given this relationship, youth workers' experiences of not-knowing reflect not only conflicts of professional identity but also profound crises of vocation or calling. Being called to the profession often contributes to youth workers differentiating themselves from other service providers (as reflected in youth workers' sense of themselves as outside and somehow above their peers in social work, as described earlier). Theirs is a certain task, to be performed in a certain way, because the world has called them to respond thusly. Folta (1995) has suggested that vocation or calling is defined by this sense of separation from the crowd for a specific purpose. When that purpose appears unattainable, as in moments of not-knowing, what happens to the call, to the justification for uniqueness? This may be the core of vocational crisis for youth workers in moments of not-knowing—it is a crisis of both profession and vocation.

NOTE

1. It bears noting that the pressure to know what to do in every situation is likely not universal among youth workers. For instance, discussions with British or South African youth workers might reveal a subtler understanding of the responsibility to respond, one with less attention to the expectation of supercompetence. Nonetheless, despite the potential limitations presented by its cultural context, the pressure to know (which I have called the *myth of supercompetence*) has resonated with many youth workers, including participants in this study and others with whom I have shared sections of the dissertation.

REFERENCES

Anglin, J. (2002). *Pain, normality, and the struggle for congruence: Reinterpreting residential care for children and youth.* New York: The Haworth Press.

Arieli, M. (1997). *The occupational experience of residential child and youth care workers: Caring and its discontents.* New York: The Haworth Press.

Bober, T., & Regehr, C. (2006). Strategies for reducing secondary or vicarious trauma: Do they work? *Brief Treatment and Crisis Intervention, 6,* 1–9.

Bournes, D. A. (2000). A commitment to honoring people's choices. *Nursing Science Quarterly, 13,* 18–23.

Brown, M. M. (1980). *What is home economics education*? Minneapolis, MN: Minnesota Research and Development Center for Vocational Education, Department of Vocational and Technical Education, University of Minnesota.

Cornille, T., & Meyers, T. W. (1999). Secondary traumatic stress among child protective service workers; Prevalence, severity, and predictive factors. *Traumatology, 5,* 15–31.

Figley, C. (1995). Compassion fatigue as secondary traumatic stress disorder: An overview. In C. Figley (Ed.), *Compassion fatigue: Coping with secondary traumatic stress disorder in those who treat the traumatized* (pp. 1–20). New York: Brunner/Mazel.

Figley, C. (2002). Compassion fatigue: Psychotherapists' chronic lack of self care. *Journal of Clinical Psychology/In Session: Psychotherapy in Practice, 58*, 1433–1441.

Folta, R. (1995). God's call. *Christian Nurse International, 11*(1), 7–8.

Gabriel, M. A. (1994). Group therapists and AIDS groups: An exploration of traumatic stress reactions. *GROUP, 18*, 167–176.

Garrett, C. (1999). Stress, coping, empathy, secondary traumatic stress, and burnout in healthcare providers working with HIV infected individuals. *Dissertation Abstracts International, 60/04-A*, 1329.

Hooker, C. E. (1976). Learned helplessness. *Social Work, 21*(3), 194–198.

Kelley, L. S. (1991). Struggling with going along when you do not believe. *Nursing Science Quarterly, 4*, 123–129.

Kelly, C. (1990). Professionalizing child and youth care: An overview. *Child and Youth Services, 13*, 167–176.

Lee, R. T., & Ashforth, B. E. (1996). A meta-analytic examination of the correlates of the three dimensions of job burnout. *Journal of Applied Psychology, 81*, 123–133.

Lesser, Y. (2007). Potential space: Knowing and not knowing in the treatment of traumatized children and young people. *British Journal of Social Work, 37*, 23–37.

Long, N., Wood, M., & Fecser, F. (2001). *Life space crisis intervention: Talking with students in conflict*. Austin: Pro-Ed.

Maslach, C. (1982). *Burnout, the cost of caring*. Englewood Cliffs, NJ: Prentice-Hall.

Mattingly, M. (2006). Managing occupational stress for group care personnel. *Child and Youth Services, 28*, 209–230.

McCann, L., & Pearlman, L. A. (1990). Vicarious traumatization: A framework for understanding the psychological effects of working with victims. *Journal of Traumatic Stress, 3*, 131–149.

McMullen, M. B., & Krantz, M. (1988). Burnout in day care workers: The effects of learned helplessness and self-esteem. *Child and Youth Care Quarterly, 17*, 278–280.

Mitchell, G. J., & Heidt, P. (1994). The lived experience of wanting to help another: Research with Parse's method. *Nursing Science Quarterly, 7*, 119–127.

Ord, J. (2004). Curriculum debate: The youth work curriculum as process, not as outcome and output to aid accountability. *Youth & Policy, 85*, 53–70.

Powell, D. (1990). Professionalism in the child care field: What model? *Child and Youth Services, 13*, 177–186.

Raatikainen, R. (1997). Nursing care as a calling. *Journal of Advanced Nursing, 25*, 1111–1115.

Robertson, S. (2004). The youth work curriculum. *Youth & Policy, 84*, 75–80.

Savicki, V. (2002). *Burnout across thirteen cultures: Stress and coping in child and youth care workers*. Westport, CT: Praeger.

Schein, E. (1973). *Professional education*. New York: McGraw-Hill.

Schön, D. A. (1983). *The reflective practitioner: How professionals think in action*. New York: Basic Books.

Shantall, T. (1998). A phenomenological analysis of suffering. *The International Forum for Logotherapy*, *21*, 111–120.

Shields, R. (1996). Meaning potentials of burnout in the helping professions. *The International Forum for Logotherapy*, *19*, 41–44.

Stanton, N. (2004). The youth work curriculum and the abandonment of informal education. *Youth & Policy*, *85*, 71–86.

Wittgenstein, L. (2001). *Philosophical investigations.* Malden, MA: Blackwell Publishing. (Original work published 1953)

Chapter 3

Investigating Not-Knowing: Research Methodology

SUMMARY. Phenomenology offers a unique and useful approach to understanding how people experience events or phenomena. The method is particularly instructive in exploring how youth workers experience and make sense of moments of not-knowing in the context of their professional relationships with young people. This chapter provides an introduction to phenomenological research, including its theoretical foundations and procedures. The research methods of this study, including participant recruitment, interview format, data analysis, and presentation, are included, as are the five themes associated with the experience of not knowing what to do: (a) the paralysis of stuckness, (b) features of despair, (c) humiliation and the fear of being found out, (d) questions of vocation and calling, and (e) the transition from not-knowing to knowing.

RESEARCH METHODOLOGY

Exploring how youth workers experienced moments of not-knowing requires a research methodology oriented toward questions of meaning. Born out of existential philosophy, phenomenology addresses these questions, seeking to identify and understand the features of a phenomenon as it is experienced in people's everyday lives. This chapter presents a brief description of phenomenology and provides the framework within which descriptive accounts of not-knowing were collected and analyzed in the original study. Where appropriate, reflections are also included on how the data from the original study have been received by youth workers and students of youth work in the intervening years. Despite not being reflected in the original research, these comments and reflections have nevertheless served as useful checks of resonance for the themes emerging from youth workers' experiences of not-knowing.

Finally, although research methodology seldom makes for engaging reading among practitioners, I have nonetheless encountered several youth workers (not to mention undergraduate and graduate students) since the original study was completed who have expressed an interest in understanding how interview-based interpretive research is conceptualized and conducted. In the interest of supporting youth workers' active engagement in research and theory-building, upon which our field's literature base relies, I have included much of the detailed descriptions of the original study, its design, and some of the difficulties encountered in conducting such a project.

Phenomenology

How do youth workers experience moments of not-knowing? It is a question of description and meaning, exploring the lived experiences and constructed or negotiated meanings of youth workers. Other research questions could have been asked: What is the relationship between not-knowing and negligence? What interventions or training components are most effective in reducing moments of not-knowing? I chose to approach my interest in youth workers' experiences from an interpretive frame for its attention to the lifeworld and lived experience and its interest in seeking meaning first and foremost.

The lifeworld, as the location and context for lived experience, is central to phenomenological inquiry. Phenomenology situates humans' negotiation with their environments as rooted in the concept of the lifeworld (Van Manen, 1997). The lifeworld is the site for the prereflective engagement between self and environment, the location of the sense of wonderment that characterizes pretheoretical human experience. We experience phenomena in their nonreflective states through our encounters with the lifeworld; it is the home of the ordinary, taken-for-granted part of everyday life. Husserl (1970) suggested that interrogating the lifeworld reveals certain phenomena deserving of study, and it is through descriptions of lived experience that these phenomena are investigated.

The lifeworld may be the location of phenomena, but lived experience is our point of entry to understanding them. Lived experience is by nature prereflective. It is the day-to-day encounter with the phenomena and objects in the lifeworld, without the imposition of reflective attention. This is a meaningful distinction here because the challenge of phenomenology is to strive for an understanding of experience *as lived*, not as reflected upon (Van Manen, 1997). Particularly in descriptive phenomenology, as presented by Husserl (1970; also in Cohen, Kahn, & Steeves, 2000), the phenomenologist strives to come close enough to the primal experience of the phenomenon to find in it the essence of the experience itself. In order to do this, it is critical that the experience be described in its concrete groundedness. By exploring descriptions of its embodied existence (without abstraction or reflection), the researcher allows the essence of the thing to reveal itself.

Heidegger (1962) and Gadamer (1976), departing from pure descriptive phenomenology, argued instead for an understanding of people's interpretations of their lived experiences. This is not to say that their hermeneutic phenomenology relies any less on the concreteness of the lived experience but, rather, that Heidegger and Gadamer orient their analyses toward understanding the meaning of the experience to the experiencer, rather than its essential structure (Cohen et al., 2000). This form of phenomenology attends at once to the experience and to the experiencing of it, emphasizing that the phenomenon is created anew by each person living it. This existential phenomenological approach is well suited to an exploration of youth workers' experiences of *self* in moments of not-knowing.

Descriptions of lived experience can be given a number of forms, each of which calls attention to a different component of the experience-as-lived. Van Manen (1997) has identified four *existentials* (or dimensions of lived experience) central to lived experience: temporal experience (how time is lived), spatial experience (how distance and space are lived), corporeal experience (how physical body is lived), and relational experience (lived experience through relationship).

The meaning or possible meanings of the phenomenon can be extracted by soliciting descriptions of a given phenomenon while being attentive to the breadth of how that experience is lived. Given the interest in understanding the meanings of not-knowing both *as it is lived* and *as it is interpreted*, existential or hermeneutic phenomenology was an appropriate research methodology for this study.

Phenomenology seeks meaning, referring to the way people understand their world as "real and significant" (Van Manen, 2000). Phenomenology holds that this search for meaning, for the understanding of phenomena, is fundamentally bound to the subjective engagement of both the participants and the researcher with their environments. The focus of study is the meaning of the phenomenon as it is experienced and the meaning of self in moments of the experience. My interest is not in identifying the factors that contribute to situations of not-knowing, nor in deriving a formula to predict conditions that create it. On the contrary, this study seeks to make clear the *meanings* of not-knowing as experienced by youth workers. Closely linked to interpretive phenomenology, the research question encouraged youth workers to attend to both their experiences of the phenomenon of not-knowing and their remembered (and at times reflected) experiences of themselves living that phenomenon. Put another way, the study emphasized the interaction between self and environment, suggesting that youth workers' experiences of not-knowing involved both an encounter with the phenomenon and a process of understanding that encounter. The interview questions and data analysis attended at once to the described and reflected narratives of self in situations of not-knowing.

Participant Recruitment

Given their emphasis on questions of human experience, all forms of interpretive research demand careful consideration to the selection of participants. For phenomenological research, with its attention to lived encounters with phenomena, it is essential to involve youth workers capable of sharing specific and concrete experiences of the phenomenon under study. In some cases, this can present a significant limitation to the method; after all, not all people who have experienced a phenomenon worth studying can articulately describe what they experienced. Fortunately, in a field that relies upon workers' abilities to elicit narratives from clients while using story and anecdote to build relationships, this limitation is less pronounced. Since the study's primary interest lay in understanding how youth workers experience moments of not-knowing, identifying participants who could isolate and describe at least one such experience became the primary recruitment concern.

The field of youth work is broad and encompasses several subfields, including religious youth work, mental health counseling, street work, work in drop-in and after-school centers, residential care, and more. The primary concern was finding youth workers who had stories to tell and expressed an interest in sharing them, and involving workers from a wide range of youth work environments provided a certain degree of additional depth to the analysis, offering a series of snapshots into how not-knowing is experienced differently (and similarly) across a number of environments. Since the completion of the initial study, stories collected from participants in workshops, in-service trainings, academic presentations, university classes, and informal conversations have provided still further insight into the range of environments in which youth workers encounter moments of not-knowing. In phenomenological terms, this reinforced my understanding that the experience is, in fact, a phenomenon commonly encountered in the youth worker's lifeworld.

The initial recruitment plan involved advertising the study through flyers and E-mail contacts in nonprofit organizations serving youth in three large cities (two in Minnesota and one in Oregon) and two medium-sized cities (one in Oregon and the other in Washington). At each step of the way, all participants and potential participants were ensured that neither their managers nor any other contact people at any given agency would be informed of their decision to (or not to) participate in the study. Given the power of shame and the fear of exposure accompanying experiences of not-knowing, this reassurance was essential, particularly in geographically small or tight-knit youth work communities.

In addition to recruitment via flyers, youth-serving nonprofit organizations whose staff might have interest in participating were contacted with a request for an in-person recruitment presentation. Through follow-up with these agencies' directors and managers, information sessions were arranged to inform staff of the research opportunity. Typically, these sessions occurred as part of the agency's or program's regular staff meeting, and participation in them ranged from 5 to 15 youth workers. These meetings presented the underlying rationale for the study, outlined the requirements of participation, and provided an opportunity for youth workers to ask questions about the research.

At times, gaining access to staff meetings was harder than others. For instance, at one large youth service agency, I encountered resistance from my first contact, the executive director. Although interested in the idea of my study, she was more concerned about the direct benefit to her organization. Upon hearing that there was no direct compensation to the agency, she denied permission for me to present my proposal to her staff but suggested that she would pass on my informational flyer (as long as it was clear to her staff that their time would *not* be compensated by the agency). In another case, I encountered and negotiated a series of administrative barriers between the direct service youth workers and me. I met first with the executive director, who then suggested I meet with the full group of program managers. Of the eight program managers present, four invited me to meet with their direct line staff. Only at these meetings did I actually encounter potential participants. Despite these difficulties, the reactions of youth workers in the field were encouraging; in nearly every information session, someone approached me with a smile, nod of the head, and a story to share. Not all became participants in the study, but their positive reactions and obvious interest in the study bolstered my sometimes-flagging spirits during this phase.

After they indicated their interest in participating in the study and had been screened for inclusion, youth workers were asked to select a location for their first interview, being attentive to their needs for comfort and familiarity, as well as issues of privacy and confidentiality. Participants were asked the number of years they had been working in the field, the sector of youth work they identified themselves as operating within, and a pseudonym by which they would be called for the duration of the study. All participants were over age 18, identified themselves as youth workers consistent with the criteria identified previously (voluntary and youth-directed work with young people, in which some significant component of the work is oriented toward teaching and learning), and had experienced at least one moment of not-knowing in relation to their work with young people. In all, 12 youth workers participated in the initial study.

Nearly all (10 out of 12) the participants were female, which reflects the sex division in the field. Ten identified as White, which may be a feature of racial distribution in the geographic regions in which the initial research took place. It may also say something about the racial breakdown of the field more generally. Participants came from mental health, homeless and street outreach, independent living skills, residential care, gay, lesbian, bisexual, and transgender (GLBT) drop-in centers, and recreational care facilities. They ranged from very new in the field (less than 3 years) to quite experienced (more than 20 years), from fairly young (25 years old) to mid-career (mid-40s), and from undergraduate through graduate education (in social work, counseling psychology, recreational education, and related disciplines). It is important to note this demographic breakdown not to demonstrate a representative sampling of the youth worker population but to illustrate the breadth of experience and background of people who experience the phenomenon of not-knowing.

Participant Interviews

In-depth, semistructured conversational interviews served as the primary text for this study. Although Van Manen (1997) has suggested that hermeneutic phenomenological analysis is often strengthened by the introduction of outside perspectives (from literature, myth, film, and the like) on the phenomenon, these interviews and their analysis matched more closely with Giorgi's (1997) descriptive phenomenology and align well with the interpretive model of analysis presented by Barritt, Beekman, Bleeker, and Mulderij (1984). Their model suggests that the researcher remain close to the texts themselves, analyzing each story individually, listening for those themes from the narrative that seem most important to the reader. These important elements, those that "fly up like sparks" (p. 5) to the reader, are then listed and analyzed across interviews, to see which are shared among narratives and how they are described similarly or differently. This approach allowed some flexibility in interpretation while still keeping the participants' stories in closest focus.

Youth workers in the study participated in one interview, ranging in length from one to two hours, in which they were invited to describe their experiences of not-knowing in the context of their work. Although the interviews maintained some general structure (see Appendix A for an example of the interview guide), their conversational nature allowed participants to take charge of the encounter. Mitchell and Heidt (1994) have suggested that this dialogical engagement (my outline with the youth workers' direction) occurs when the narrator or participant and researcher negotiate the direction and pace of the interview. Throughout I strove to reach this negotiated balance between me and the participants. In most cases, it was clearly established, as youth workers settled into a balance of comfortable storytelling and deliberate engagement with the central research questions.

As described above, youth workers chose a location for the interview where they felt comfortable, where confidentiality could be assured, and where the conversation could flow without likelihood of interruption. We met in youth workers' homes, in agency meeting rooms, in public parks, and in the meeting rooms of public libraries. In each case, the participants were familiar with the environment and most often positioned themselves as hosts to me, which contributed to setting a tone of comfort and dialogue.

Not-knowing is difficult for many people to talk about, particularly in a field where we are encouraged to see this experience as illustrative of our own professional failing or incompetence. With that in mind, I was conscious of participants' potential emotional discomfort throughout the interviews. In many cases, as noted in the transcripts, youth workers became emotionally invested in the stories they told: their speech patterns became more rapid, their body language changed, and, in some cases, they even became teary. In nearly every case, however, participants mentioned at the end of the interview that they felt a sense of relief at having the opportunity to share their stories and unload some of the built-up emotion surrounding them.

ANALYZING THE DATA

After each interview, I reviewed my written notes (taken during the interview and typically consisting of little more than behavioral observation and one-word cues noting key phrases to be explored later in the interview) and transcribed the tape of the session. In most cases, the transcriptions were completed within 48 hours of the interview to preserve important details of the interview that might otherwise be lost or forgotten (gestures, facial features, etc.).

Several techniques exist for the analysis of phenomenological text, from Giorgi's (1997) rather formal descriptive orientation to Van Manen's (1997) more hermeneutic approach. This study assumed a middle-of-the-road stance that remains as close as possible to the text as written while also letting the text speak for itself and allowing themes to emerge. This approach has been presented by Barritt et al. (1984) and is informed by the philosophical work of Heidegger (1962) and Gadamer (1976). The analysis itself consisted of several phases, beginning with writing first about associations and assumptions abut the phenomenon (with the intent of purging these preconceptions before approaching the text) and continuing through individual and cross-interview analysis.

Individual (Vertical) Analysis

I began my text analysis with several careful reads of each interview individually and on its own merit. I approached each read with a different goal. Initially, each interview was read twice to become familiar with the overall tone and the youth worker's word choices and phrasing. Next, the text was examined with attention to the flow and structure of the interview, outlining the main segments or chunks of the participant's narrative. On the next read, key descriptive words or phrases were identified and probed in explanatory notes in the left-hand column of the transcript. Finally, the interview and my notes were read together, with attention to the subtlety and nuance of language and representation in each. The primary interest here was to ensure that the notes were reflective of both the tone and the significant sections of text that emerged as illustrative of the experience of self in moments of not-knowing. I compiled these illustrative phrases into lists of significant elements; Barritt et al. (1984) refer to them as *forms* of the experience. Each form was accompanied by excerpts of the actual language youth workers used to describe that portion of their experience. In some cases, elements seemed related but still somewhat distinct, even after several reads of the same section of text. In these cases, the slight variations and their associated descriptive phrases were included in the list of forms.

The themes and notes from each interview were then used to draft individual interview summaries consisting of three sections: a narrative summary, a thematic summary, and general notes and key phrases. The narrative summary included my general thoughts about the interview, about the themes emerging from the preliminary analysis, and about how these themes might fit (or contrast) with other participants' descriptions. This summary was at once a recap of the interview and a preliminary dialogue across interviews. This served as parts-whole-parts (Gadamer, 1976) dialogue with the immediate text and the larger context of the study, which allows the findings to be understood and interpreted as they stand alone and as they relate to one another and the emerging whole.

Each thematic summary highlighted and commented on the forms emerging from the interview. Using the youth workers' own language where possible, I presented the form and commented on its meaning to me as the hearer of the experience. The purpose of the thematic summary was twofold: it provided an opportunity to engage in some depth with the forms while also generating a narrative to send back to the youth worker as a check of resonance, which serves as the primary source of validity for interpretive research.

The final section, including notes and key phrases, served as a condensed version of the interview transcript. It provided an index of the key concepts and descriptions of the forms in the participants' own words, along with some interpretive groupings and notations. This condensed collection of key phrases essentially functions as a quick, visual reminder of the key phrases (and links to specific pages and quotes in the transcript itself) to be used in generating a full thematic analysis table.

The youth workers themselves were directly involved in the last stage of the individual analysis. Via E-mail, I returned to them their thematic summaries (in some cases I also sent the narrative summary). I asked them to review the forms for their resonance: Did my interpretation match with the way they lived the experience? Did I misunderstand or misrepresent anything in my interpretation? Resonance of this sort is one of the hallmarks of good interpretive research, and without the participants' ultimate approval, any interpretations of mine would be inadequate. With few exceptions, participants reported high levels of satisfaction and resonance with my interpretations. In those few exceptional cases, the participants' clarifications were integrated into the analysis.

Thematic (Horizontal) Analysis

Phenomenological research would be useless if it failed to provide a deep understanding of an experience or a phenomenon shared across the rich descriptions of many individuals with first-hand accounts of the experience—whether through interviews, written narratives, or other sources. Of course, the volume of text generated by collecting these descriptions can make the task of sifting through the data to find meaningful connections a difficult one. In some cases, narratives can yield several hundred pages of material to be analyzed.

In order to reduce youth workers' descriptions from individual summary to common theme, I drew from Barritt et al. (1984), using an analysis table to identify themes. With each participant as a column and each row as a theme, the significant forms for each interview were listed in the table. Looking horizontally across the table identified themes that appeared to resonate consistently (even if in varied forms) across the youth workers' descriptions. The table also helped to facilitate the back-and-forth between the descriptive and interpretive elements of phenomenological research, balancing the participants' descriptions of their experiences with my own interpretation of their meaning.

The challenge of analyzing and interpreting these narratives involves identifying strands that run through the descriptive text and teasing out which are essential to the experience. These essential themes are then explored and plumbed for their own depth. Throughout the entire process, the researcher returns again and again from the theme to the whole body of narrative descriptions collected during the research phase: How are the themes related to the overall tone of the data collected? How do they relate to one another? What has been overlooked in identifying the themes? What might have been exaggerated?

These questions led to the identification of variations within the thematic groupings. While themes are general, variations provide subtlety and texture. Each variation offers a different take on the general direction of the theme, providing additional depth and richness to the description of the experience or phenomenon. Throughout the study, the term *variation* refers to the diverse manifestations of a theme. The term is not to be confused with the practice of imaginative variation evident in many phenomenological analyses. For these purposes, variations are better understood as subtleties than alternatives—they demonstrate the depth of the theme rather than deviations from it. Since not all phenomena are experienced in the same way, variations function as illustrations of the diversity found in narrative descriptions of a phenomenon's dominant features. Consider the parable of the blind men and the elephant. Although all the men touch the same elephant, one (at the leg) describes the object as thick and hard, like a tree stump. Another, at the ear, experiences the elephant as smooth, thin, and broad, like a kite. The third, touching the elephant's side, says the object is as big as a house and rough in texture. All are touching the same elephant, and all descriptions are accurate; they are merely different expressions of the object.

Having compiled lists of forms, themes, variations, and statements, each theme was then interrogated to determine whether it was essential to the experience. I encountered themes that initially appeared to be essential but which on further investigation and theorizing revealed themselves to be variations on larger themes. Holding these elements in conversation with the dominant themes was essential in developing my final interpretation and generating the composite experiences of youth workers' experiences of not-knowing-what-to-do.

ORGANIZING AND PRESENTING THE DATA

Several themes describing how youth workers experienced not-knowing came into view for me after spending several months with nearly 30 hours of narrative interview text. These themes have been reinforced by many additional hours in consultation with youth workers in a number of environments since the completion of the study. In the process of distilling and interrogating these themes, I found that the lines between some blurred while others sharpened. Some themes that appeared clear at the beginning of my analysis revealed themselves to be, instead, variations on still other themes. Eventually, five general themes (with their associated variations) emerged as illustrative of youth workers' experiences of not-knowing:

Theme 1: Like a deer in the headlights: The paralysis of stuckness
Variations: It's just me, and that's not enough
It's like a mental freefall
That crushing becomes your world

Theme 2: Helpless, hopeless, and out of control: Features of despair
Variations: There was nothing there to protect me
Something else just took control of everything
What does he have to do, kill someone?!

Theme 3: Center stage: Humiliation, being found out, and the myth of supercompetence
Variations: The worst public humiliation
They'll know I'm a fraud

Theme 4: It's just a little too human: Questions of vocation
Variations: What am I supposed to do?
Who am I to deal with this?
Maybe the problem is me

Theme 5: Not-knowing gives way to knowing
Variations: Annie! Annie! Are you okay? The rousing power of someone else
I have to respond, because there's no one else
The power of winging it

Identifying the themes and variations is only part of analysis. As suggested in previous chapters, there are several traditions of phenomenological interpretation and analysis. With regard to interpretation and presentation of themes, the descriptive phenomenology advanced by Giorgi (1997) suggests that the researcher should remain as close to the narrative descriptions as possible, introducing few additional external sources and limiting the role of the researcher's own interpretive sense. Van Manen's (1997) hermeneutic approach, in contrast, emphasizes the role of interpretation and application on the part of the researcher. Resonance, the hallmark of good phenomenological research, is facilitated by looking for similar or particularly poignant and complementary descriptions between the narrative text and works of literature, art, or even the interpreter's own experiences.

In analyzing how youth workers describe their moments of not-knowing, I drew generously from both traditions without fully committing to either. Throughout the process, it was important to me to allow the workers' stories to speak freely and to illustrate the central themes of their experiences. Believing in the explanatory and descriptive power of their own words, I wanted to present each youth worker's story without smothering them with my external interpretive lens. After all, the need to hear these stories and their meaning from one another, normalizing the experience in the process, is what brought me to the project in the first place.

Nonetheless, at the same time, I wanted to attend to the meaning of these descriptions, an effort for which the hermeneutic tradition is of some help. Gadamer (1976) has suggested that experiences or phenomena can be best understood in the context of the experiencers' own interpretations. This position encourages the active integration of the narrators' lived descriptions *and* their reflected-upon interpretations of those experiences. This interpretive tradition, informed by Gadamer and presented by Barritt et al. (1984), bridged the descriptive and hermeneutic positions. Adopting this stance helped me to see two distinct groups of themes, one largely descriptive and the other more interpretive, in the narratives.

The first category, consisting of the first three themes, deals with the individual and distinct features of youth workers' experiences as they lived them. These themes are richly descriptive, relating primarily to the lived experience of the moment of not-knowing. They attend to what it was like, physically, spatially, temporally, and relationally (Van Manen, 1997) for youth workers to experience the moment of not-knowing. Although the details of the events of not-knowing differed widely, these three themes ran consistently through the narratives. Focusing almost completely on how youth workers experienced lived body, space, and time in the moment of not-knowing (and very little on what meaning they made of these experiences after the fact), this grouping is more purely descriptive than interpretive. Identifying the features of the experience captured in these themes can help youth workers recognize features of not-knowing as they emerge in future situations, which may alleviate some of the intensity, self-criticism, and vocational crisis often accompanying such moments.

The second group, themes four and five, probes deeper into how youth workers reflect on their moments of not-knowing during and after the experience itself. In these themes, youth workers described the meanings they made of not-knowing when they were most conscious of it. Also richly descriptive, these themes contain more interpretation than pure lived experience. They present the struggles or comforts youth workers encountered in confronting the meaning of not-knowing and attend to the vocational and professional questions that follow. These themes point toward the questions and dilemmas facing youth work as a field, identifying issues in need of ongoing professional training, awareness, and open discourse.

More than anything else, in presenting the emergent themes of not-knowing, I wanted to ensure that both the situations giving rise to them and the experiences of the youth workers themselves were conveyed with sensitivity and honesty. It was essential, in my mind, that the themes be presented in context, as they were (or could have been) lived, and that the presentation itself resonated with other youth workers' experiences.

With this in mind and in the tradition of hermeneutic phenomenology, each of the five themes is introduced in subsequent chapters by a composite story of a moment of not-knowing. These composites, although partially fictionalized, are built from features of several different youth workers' experiences and contain, in many cases, the very phrases used in individual interviews. In contrast to the actual experience of not-knowing, which may involve elements of several themes at once, I wrote each vignette to highlight the central characteristics and variations of a single theme. These narrative stories introduce each theme, after which I provide a more detailed exploration of the theme and its variations, as I heard them from the participants and interpreted them through my own lenses as both researcher and fellow youth worker.

The characters in each of the vignettes are fictionalized, although in many places, they closely resemble actual youth workers. Using the vignettes as additional narratives, I wove descriptions from the actual stories through the interpretations. In order to ensure, again, that the composites were both believable and illustrative of their corresponding themes, I conducted another resonance check on each. Having stripped them of any identifying information, I sent each composite to colleagues in the field, youth workers in direct practice who did *not* participate in the study, with the following questions: Is this situation realistic? What themes do you hear in this narrative? Additional clarifications or suggestions were incorporated into the final vignettes.

REFERENCES

Barritt, L., Beekman, T., Bleeker, H., & Mulderij, K. (1984). Analyzing phenomenological descriptions. *Phenomenology & Pedagogy*, *2*, 1–17.

Cohen, M. Z., Kahn, D. L., & Steeves, R. H. (2000). *Hermeneutic phenomenological research: A practical guide for nurse researchers*. Thousand Oaks, CA: Sage.

Gadamer, H. G. (1976). *Philosophical hermeneutics* (D. E. Linge, Ed. & Trans.). Berkeley: University of California Press.

Giorgi, A. (1997). The theory, practice and evaluation of the phenomenological method as a qualitative research procedure. *Journal of Phenomenological Psychology*, *28*, 235–260.

Heidegger, M. (1962). *Being and time* (J. Macquarrie & E. Robinson, Trans.). New York: Harper & Row.

Husserl, E. (1970). *The crisis of European sciences and transcendental phenomenology*. Evanston: Northwestern University Press.

Mitchell, G. J., & Heidt, P. (1994). The lived experience of wanting to help another: Research with Parse's method. *Nursing Science Quarterly*, *7*, 119–127.

Van Manen, M. (1997). *Researching lived experience: Human science for an action sensitive pedagogy* (2nd ed.). London, Ontario: Althouse.

Van Manen, M. (2000). *Glossary*. Retrieved May 12, 2003, from Phenomenology Online Web site: www.phenomenologyonline.com/glossary.cfm?range=All# lived%20meaning.

Chapter 4

Whose Stories *are* These?

SUMMARY. Phenomenological research investigates the meaning of lived experiences for participants, as well as the implications of those experiences. This chapter presents brief biographical sketches of 12 youth workers who participated in a phenomenological investigation of the experience of self in moments of not-knowing what to do. Each participant's characteristics, professional location in the broad field of American youth work, and circumstances surrounding the experience of not-knowing are described.

WHO ARE THE PARTICIPANTS?

I was contacted by many youth workers who expressed interest in participating in the original study. The 12 whose narratives ultimately provided the text for this exploration of not-knowing shared experiences that were both insightful and painful. Tears were shed during many of our interviews, and laughter was a feature of them all. In each interview (and each of the follow-up conversations between me and the youth workers in the original study), I was struck by the participants' openness and honesty. They all wanted their stories to be told, they all believed in this project, and they all trusted that their experiences would speak to and help link them with other youth workers struggling in our field. The stories of these 12 people not only built the foundation for the original study but also shaped my subsequent discussions of not-knowing with other audiences. By their willingness to share their moments, these youth workers have given permission for others to do the same.

In telling a story, they unknowingly set the stage for colleagues they never met to tell theirs as well. They are not simply research participants. They are narrators of experience. Edwards (2000) uses this title, narrators, to describe participants in interpretive research. It is a useful term for the participants in this project. Their voices have shaped, explained, and summarized the not-knowing experience for the broader youth work audience. At the same time, however, we cannot allow their narration to be merely a detached, faceless voice-over, safely separated from the text. They have been my partners in crafting this work from the very beginning, and although features of their individual stories run through the composites that introduce the coming chapters, they each deserve their own spotlight here. It is my hope, as it was theirs, that these brief sketches of each participant helps bring them to life for readers, and that this in turn helps youth workers see themselves more clearly in this text.

Athena

Athena has worked in the field for many years and holds a master's degree in social work. She chose Athena, Greek goddess of wisdom and battle, as her pseudonym—adding that the name suits her orientation to her work. She carries herself as an ally to youth in a world where affirming youth as full, complete, competent beings is often a battle against structures that deny them. Athena strives for the wisdom and introspection to sustain her in this battle. She is a deeply spiritual woman, possessed of a calm warmth that sets the most wary and defensive of people at ease. She is joyful and laughs easily, while also being sensitive and quick to cry when she sees others in pain. Most of her work has taken place with homeless and street youth in a major urban center, although she has also worked extensively with pregnant and parenting teens in independent living programs.

We met at a sidewalk coffee shop on a warm summer day, and Athena shared two clear moments of not-knowing. The first involved an overt act of racism committed in a very public place by a White woman against one of Athena's clients, a young Black teen mother. Although the client had done nothing wrong, beyond allowing her child to play and giggle during a cartoon movie, she was insulted with racist epithets and veiled physical threats by a total stranger, a White woman two decades older than she. It was a situation that struck Athena not only because of the overt nature of the encounter but also because although it took place in public (in front of a movie theater), no passersby attempted to intervene. Despite her own rage at the injustice and empathy for her client, Athena found herself paralyzed, unable to respond.

Her second story was about her relationship with a young gay man in a drop-in center who struggled to integrate his sexual orientation with his family's strong evangelical Christian values and statements of rejection from his caregivers. The height of not-knowing occurred when the young man looked at Athena and asked, with tears in his eyes, "Do you think God still loves me?"

Cleve

Cleve has been involved in youth services in a small city for more than 10 years. In the community, she is known as a powerful school interventionist and skilled practitioner. Her peers and clients alike also talk about her somewhat crass humor, her ability to laugh at herself, and her fierce dedication to her work. Her background in community- and school-based youth work has given her considerable exposure to the impact of mental health, child protection, juvenile justice, and child placement services on young people.

Our interview took place in a park Cleve had chosen, which gave the conversation a relaxed and comfortable tone. Over the course of our 2-hour conversation, Cleve shared experiences of not-knowing that came from her interactions with other professionals while attempting to advocate on behalf of youth in multi-systems team meetings. Few of her moments of stuckness related to working directly with youth; she said that she's become increasingly comfortable accepting these experiences as they happen. Instead, she told of feeling silenced and shamed by other professionals and highlighted the fear of being exposed as a fraud due to what other social service staff perceived to be her inadequate (bachelor's-level) education. In both cases, Cleve was most aware of not-knowing what to do in terms of balancing her own emotional responses with the immediate needs of her clients.

Drizzt

One of only two male participants, Drizzt has worked in the community mental health system for about 5 years. Initially drawn to working with youth in this system out of a desire to simply be helpful to people in need, he has struggled with the programmatic and administrative barriers that often interfere with the delivery of the very services they are intended to facilitate. His frustration with these systems, at the same time that he continues to work within them, is clear when Drizzt talks. It is fitting that he chose his pseudonym in honor of a fiercely independent and passionate character from a fantasy novel.

On the day we met in his office's group room, sitting together on couches surrounded by plants, Drizzt talked about the fatigue associated with the demands of his work, attempting to provide services to too many young people with too few resources. Drizzt's experience of not-knowing formed the basis, in many ways, of the vignette that introduces the theme of futility and despair. He told of sitting with the family of a seriously disturbed client and being begged by the mother to provide a service intervention that his agency's policies and funding requirements prevented him from providing. He told me that the moment of not-knowing was most pronounced for him when his client's mother looked to him with tears in her eyes and asked, "What does he have to do [to get help], kill someone?!" Forced to simply stare at this mother, with no response and no resources to offer, Drizzt struggled to justify his continued role in a helping system that is often completely unable to help.

Eve

Eve was one of the few participants in the study who had left the field by the time of our interview. Although during our interview there were moments during which I wondered whether she regretted the decision, it was clear that she needed to tell her story. When she had initially contacted me, she asked—almost apologetically—if she could still participate. At our interview, she told me she had hoped to be able to be included in the study because she wanted the chance to talk, finally, about some of the events that led her to leave youth work. As her story unfolded, I was struck by her calm, soothing demeanor and deliberate attention to words, choosing her phrases and images carefully, even in relating painful events that still held a significant emotional charge.

We met in a study room at a neighborhood branch of her large city's public library system. In a voice that was both quiet and strong—even when sharing events she experienced as punishing—Eve talked about one specific experience of not-knowing as the last in a long series of events that ultimately led to her leaving youth work. Her moment of not-knowing took place in a group home for young adult men who had been labeled emotionally or behaviorally disordered and were considered unsafe to continue living with their families. Eve's experience centered around one afternoon, when a young man with whom she had worked for months joined with another resident in verbally attacking her. Initially unable to move herself out of the situation, Eve stood in place and felt herself collapsing under a barrage of insults and slurs. Although she recognized that these kinds of episodes were commonplace in the facility and that they held the potential to be significant therapeutic opportunities for intervention, Eve found herself unable to respond. She described being overwhelmed by their verbal assault, losing control of herself altogether and physically fleeing from the room, ultimately leaving the job within a matter of weeks.

Lily

Sitting in the living room of her comfortable home a few miles outside the medium-sized city where she lives and works, Lily provided a rich and detailed description of not-knowing from an interaction with a young person earlier that same day. I was immediately impressed with her storytelling. Lily speaks with a clarity that is almost piercing, demonstrating a high level of introspection and willingness to analyze her own experiences, searching for the learning they might possess. Her experience struck me at the time as significant largely because, for so many youth workers, it is common to the point of being almost not worth discussing. The power of the experience is its ability to illustrate that not all moments of not-knowing occur in dramatic, crisis-oriented settings. At times, the very discussion that bored us on Wednesday can paralyze us on Friday.

Working with young people to develop independent and transitional living skills, Lily talked about the frustration and stuckness she experienced with a client who simply would not take responsibility for following through on tasks essential for her continued participation in the agency's services. Despite all the creative intervention and engagement strategies Lily tried, this client simply would not follow through. Although not a crisis situation, there was, nevertheless, a sense of urgency to the interaction, since this was not a client Lily could see being able to function without her program's support, and she was on the edge of being removed from the program as noncompliant. Lily talked about the physical and mental paralysis she experienced in the height of not-knowing, staring blankly at her client with no idea how to move the situation beyond this stuck place.

Lori

Still somewhat new to the field, Lori has worked as a counselor and case manager in an urban drop-in center for gay, lesbian, bisexual, transgender, and queer youth for the past couple of years. Interpersonally, she has the energy of a drop-in worker: eager to engage, outgoing, and friendly. It was easy to imagine Lori welcoming youth into an unfamiliar space, helping them feel at ease, and quickly forming the youth-staff relationships that emerge uniquely in milieu settings like the drop-in.

We met in the drop-in center during off-hours and shared a cup of coffee as Lori talked about her experience of not knowing what to do. Her story involved coming to work and hearing that a client whom she knew very well and with whom she shared a strong emotional bond was dying in a city more than two states away. Trying to manage her own emotional response, questions, and exhaustion while being attentive to the needs of the other youth in the center (most of whom knew the young man, as well), Lori became conscious of having no idea how to respond. It broke her heart, she said, that she could not be helpful to the youth in the way she wanted; she could not take their pain away (nor could she fully experience her own). She shared a second story, as well, of trying to help a client whose depression bordered on suicidal but who would not consent to intervention. Lori spent several hours in her office working with this young woman and finally had to allow her client to walk out of the center, with no idea whether or not she would return the next day. Similar to Lily, the fear of what could happen to the youth in the absence of the program and supports it offered became paralyzing.

Martin

Martin works in homeless and street youth outreach in the same small city where he began his career 20 years ago. He is a soft-spoken but charismatic man who prefers to spend his time on the street working with detached and mistrusting youth rather than in the office or conference room at his agency. Martin is introspective and clever, with a quick wit and a funny little sparkle in his eye. It is easy to see, immediately, what makes him so effective at engaging young people.

We met at Martin's dining room table on an incredibly warm summer afternoon, and he talked generally about his reflections on the field, the challenges he encounters in doing youth work, and some of the specific moments he has experienced not knowing what to do. The first story Martin shared involved a crisis incident at a coed group home early in his career. He had given permission for a young man to go unsupervised to help someone fix a stalled car and was surprised by a loud "boom," and the same young man running up the driveway to the group home, covered in battery acid. Torn between attending to this client and responding to the several other youth standing nearby, Martin felt momentarily stuck in the moment of not-knowing. He shared a second story that mirrors Lily's and Lori's in many ways, describing the frustration and futility of not knowing what to do after trying to provide services to a young person who refused to follow through on his obligations but lacked the skills to succeed without these services.

Ophelia

Ophelia has worked with youth in her small city for 8 years. She is a funny woman who often laughs, as often at herself as at a shared joke. She recently finished a master's degree and hopes to use her continued education to support young people in a community where social services are often difficult to come by—an observation that causes her eyes to become teary when we discuss it. We met in one of her agency's conference rooms for nearly 2 hours, as she related a poignant and emotionally charged experience of being with a young client and his mother in a consultation appointment with another professional, when the boy suddenly and without provocation attacked. First, he attacked his mother, rushing her from the other side of the room and starting to hit and claw at her face. Within seconds, he turned and began rushing and attacking Ophelia. She described her paralysis in the moment, not knowing how to respond to the situation, coupled with her frustration that, despite graduate training and years of experience, she could still be so shocked by a client's behavior.

The end of Ophelia's story involved her reflection on the experience. She became teary and her voice shook as she talked about the grief associated with working on behalf of people who are so emotionally fragile and raw, while unable to find the appropriate support for them. Hers became one of the central stories, along with Athena, Vanessa, and Lori, of futility as it is experienced in the moment of not-knowing.

Stella

Stella impressed me from the first E-mail she sent me. In writing and in person, she comes across as a powerful and engaging woman, quick with stories and eager to engage new people. With a background in the arts, Stella speaks in metaphor and imagery, drawing clear pictures of her experiences. Although it was at times hard for her to describe in words what the moment of not-knowing was like for her, the metaphors she chose brought me into the experience as though I had shared it.

Stella and I met in a public study room at the local library. She told of an experience that occurred in a short-term shelter program for homeless and runaway youth where she had worked for a short time. It was her first youth work position, and she had left the agency some time before our meeting. At the time of our conversation, she identified herself as a youth worker but was uncertain whether she would work professionally in the field again. The experience she shared was one in which a young Latina woman came out to her, disclosing that she identified as a lesbian, and looked to Stella for advice and approval. The high point of not-knowing occurred for Stella when this client began interrogating her about her own sexual orientation. Stella felt caught between wanting to be personally and emotionally present for what this client was asking and needing to maintain the professional face demanded of her in the program. As her client's demands for self-disclosure intensified, so did the stuckness Stella identified with the experience of not knowing how to respond.

Stephanie

When Stephanie first contacted me about participation in the study, she mentioned that she was not interested in the compensation youth workers received for participating. Instead, she asked that we have a conversation after the study was completed so she could hear what I had learned and pass it along to her staff. When we actually met in person, I was immediately struck by her energy and passion for the children with whom her agency works and for the ongoing professional development of fellow youth workers. Stephanie has held a variety of youth work positions in her 10 years in the field, ranging from domestic violence education to residential work with developmentally disabled young adults. Introspection and a desire to further develop professional skill through interpersonal collaboration have been consistent threads through her career.

We met in the conference room of her agency, and Stephanie launched right into her story (which she, like several other participants) had never told for a purpose other than comic relief at dinner parties and social engagements. The not-knowing experience Stephanie shared came from early in her career, on one of her first shifts in a group home for autistic youth. She told a story of being physically attacked twice by the same client, not out of anger, but due to some cues conveyed by Stephanie's behavior that she had no way to anticipate. Unbeknownst to Stephanie, anyone crossing any part of their bodies (arms folded across one's chest, legs crossed at the knee, etc.) agitated this young woman and she felt compelled to make the behavior stop. She attacked Stephanie, raking down her bare arms with her fingernails. Stephanie described the paralysis she felt as, bleeding, she tried to make sense of what had just happened, reconcile the fact that none of the staff in the facility seemed to see anything problematic about the experience, determine how to be helpful to her client, and keep herself physically safe.

Sweet Pea

Sweet Pea works with gay, lesbian, bisexual, and transgendered young people in a major urban setting. She contacted me via E-mail in response to my recruitment materials and was excited to participate in the study. When we met in the conference room of her agency, she struck me as remarkably collected and self-confident. Although her stories carried the same tone of discomfort, fear, and embarrassment that ran through many other youth workers' narratives, Sweet Pea spoke with a powerful directness that belied any underlying insecurity or anxiety.

The first story Sweet Pea shared took place in a rural residential treatment center where she had worked at the beginning of her career. She told of being approached by two young women who were known to be in a romantic relationship and asked by them whether or not she, herself, was a lesbian. On the spot and fearful of the implications of her answer, juggling what she wanted to say with what she believed she was expected by agency policy to say, Sweet Pea had no idea how to respond. The second experience formed the basis for this study's final vignette. Sweet Pea found herself pressured by a group of youth to be allowed to jump off the cliffs at a popular swimming hole. Conscious of the potential danger but also wanting to reward the youth for their model behavior earlier in the day and allow kids to be kids, Sweet Pea was at a loss for a response. She remained stuck until pulled back into the moment by the unsolicited involvement of a complete stranger.

Vanessa

Vanessa is perhaps the most quiet and reserved of the youth workers who participated in the study. What at first struck me as shyness was, by the end of our conversation, a gentle warmth and genuine care that seems to characterize her interactions. Of all the participants, Vanessa struggled the most to identify a pseudonym, finally deciding on "Vanessa" because the name made her think of a dangerous, edgy alter ego for her generally reserved personality.

We met in a counseling room at the urban youth service agency where Vanessa has been employed for a short time. She has worked with youth in a variety of community mental health and social service settings for the past few years. She shared an experience of not-knowing that helped shape the vignette for the fourth theme, concerning questions of calling and vocation. Vanessa described a counseling session with a young man, midway through her master's degree, where she had been tasked with assessing this youth's suitability for public school and continued community living. Other members of his community support team had advocated for him to be sent to a residential program for behaviorally disturbed youth, and it was left up to Vanessa to make the final recommendation. Mindful that her impressions and recommendations would likely play a significant role in shaping the next several years of this young person's life, and conscious of her own discomfort with the power of her situation, Vanessa felt paralyzed. Feeling pressured to fix this young man, but receiving little or no investment from him, she found herself not knowing how to reconcile her discomfort with being put in the expert role with her uncertainty about her own competence and fighting the temptation to run for the hills, leaving youth work permanently.

REFERENCE

Edwards, N. (2000). *Works in progress: Ten women's transitional journeys in the realm of sexuality.* Unpublished doctoral dissertation, University of Minnesota, Twin Cities.

Chapter 5

Like a Deer in the Headlights: The Paralysis of Stuckness

SUMMARY. When describing how they experience moments of not-knowing, youth workers often talk about a sense of paralysis, as though their uncertainty becomes physically constraining. This chapter describes the first of five themes associated with youth workers' experiences of not knowing what to do: the paralysis of stuckness. In addition to describing and investigating the dominant theme of paralysis, this chapter discusses its three variations, as described by youth worker participants: (a) It's just me, and that's not enough, (b) It's like a mental freefall, and (c) That crushing becomes your world.

VIGNETTE: THE TROUBLE WITH MITCH

As soon as he walked into the drop-in, I started feeling anxious—like the knots you get in your stomach just before you get sick. Mitch had been coming to the center for quite a while, most recently with the girlfriend he said he was going to marry. That was something we, as staff at the center, were all nervous about; it was pretty clear that Mitch was abusive toward her. He had a short fuse with everyone, but he kept Danielle on a particularly tight leash. It wasn't at all uncommon for Danielle to come to the center with bruises on her arms and face and all sorts of elaborate explanations of how she had gotten them.

Today, though, Mitch came in alone, cutting straight through the crowd of other kids in the center, in search of Danielle. When he found out she wasn't there, he started cussing a blue streak and calling her a whore. He said she was making him look like a chump and needed to be taught a lesson. The other staff and I looked at each other, sharing one of those "this is going to be a problem" looks. It was clear that we needed to separate and deescalate Mitch in order to keep the main drop-in space safe. Since I was the only male present, I tried to draw him away from the rest of the youth. I remember thinking right then that I was in over my head, but I figured it was one of those sink-or-swim, baptism-by-fire moments.

I was already scared as we sat down together in the counseling room, which was just off the main room of the center. I had no idea what was supposed to happen next. Even as mad as he was, I don't think I was worried about him hitting me, but I didn't know what I was going to do to calm him down, either. It felt urgent, though. I knew that if he *didn't* calm down, Danielle (at least) was going to wind up hurt. Palms sweating, I started racing through my mental toolbox, trying to find the right intervention to get the situation under control. I tried everything I could think of, every intervention I had been taught, but nothing seemed to work. I was at a loss.

The whole process felt really disorienting. I didn't know what I could possibly do to make the situation any better, but I knew I had to do *something*. I felt overwhelmed and alone. I could just barely hear the other youth in the center talking about him, and somewhere in the back of my head, I knew that if I heard them, Mitch probably could also. Would that make him go off even more? Hearing them on the other side of the wall made me feel that much more isolated on my side of it. I wanted someone to come rescue me, because he was escalating and nothing I tried was working. Mitch kept getting angrier and angrier, and his words came faster and louder. I was completely overwhelmed—I didn't know what I could do to deal with this situation. I didn't think there was anything I *could* do any more. My grip on reality was just slipping away.

Then I remember hearing commotion in the other room; Danielle had come into the center. I felt panicked. My energy was out of control, totally wild, but at the same time, I couldn't really move or even *think* straight. I was scrambling, frantic, totally out of control of the situation and my own body. What do we do now? What do *I* do now, in here, with him? We were all in too deep, but the other staff had each other. I was by myself! There wasn't anyone else—just me. There was no help coming. It was just what I, *personally*, had to go by. I was flying blind. And that wasn't going to be enough.

I felt completely fragmented—like half my mind was out in the other room watching Danielle, and the other half was still in the room with Mitch, trying to keep him there. I didn't have one whole mind to deal with much of anything. It was really disorienting, really out-of-body, like a mental freefall. But what could I do? It was like being in a tiny boat tossed around in the middle of a storm. I remember looking around the room, searching for an anchor, something I could use to distract Mitch and get him to focus on something (anything) else. But I couldn't grab hold of anything. I was just stuck, floating. I couldn't touch down. I was stuck.

I think Mitch heard Danielle at that point, because I could see him building more steam. There wasn't anything I could do about it, though. I couldn't focus on anything other than his anger and the fact that I couldn't think of anything to make it go away. Sitting across from me, he kept puffing up, growing in his chair, and I started to feel smaller and smaller in mine. I remember thinking that this wasn't how things were supposed to go; *I* was supposed to be in charge of the situation! *I* was supposed to know how to handle things like this! But I didn't. I didn't know any of it. I was completely stuck, wrapped up in what was happening in that room, absolutely unable to move a muscle, afraid that I'd already lost control.

It was oppressive. It was like being in a dark, dense cloud. I could hear his voice, but it was muffled. I could see his movements, but they seemed slowed down and exaggerated. It was like I had shrunk down into my chair and was being crushed by the weight of the cushions, the walls, the ceiling. Everything slowed down, like I could *feel* myself thinking, but I couldn't *do* anything about it. Mitch was still there, but only kind of. It was like somebody had wrapped a pillow all the way around my head, and that pillow was just crushing in on me. I could see out, but only through this tiny little hole. It was like tunnel vision—all I could see was Mitch, but I couldn't do anything about it. My mind was blank. It was an absolute, crushing blank. There was just nothing there. Nothing but pressure and tunnel vision. And even though I was supposed to know how to handle the situation, all I could do was sit with him, watching him get more and more angry and more and more volatile.

LIKE A DEER IN THE HEADLIGHTS

Time and time again in my research, in the youth work practice classes I teach, and in everyday conversation, youth workers share descriptions of events that highlight a profound experience of physical paralysis. The moment of not-knowing is one they live physically; it is not only not-knowing but also not-being-able-to. Invoking a variety of images and comparisons, youth workers shared their awareness of their bodies, of physical space, and of how it physically felt to not know how to respond. Throughout the interview process, several youth workers found it difficult to convey their experience of not-knowing without abstraction and reflection. When they started talking about their experience of feeling stuck, however, it repeatedly struck me how easily they shared lived-body, lived-space, and lived-time stories. These descriptions were not presented in terms of an abstracted sense of inability. Rather, youth workers shared vivid and embodied descriptions of what it was like to be in their bodies at the moment when they were most aware of being stuck. In many cases, their stories came tumbling out of their mouths as though, regardless of how much they had processed the events in supervision or consultation, they had never before been presented with an opportunity to talk about what it was actually *like* to be in their skin during those events.

Although the circumstances in which they arose differed widely, descriptions of physical paralysis as a defining feature of not-knowing grouped tightly around three images: isolation, anchorlessness, and pressure. For many, not-knowing was connected to a sense of isolation and bodily alienation. This was not merely an awareness of being by oneself; it is better likened to the experience of having no one and nothing to look toward for support, guidance, or sympathy. It included the panicked paralysis that comes with the recognition that one is not only alone but also completely lost.

Others described their paralysis as being out-of-body. In this variation, youth workers talked about a floating sensation, one in which they had no foundation, no grounding. Feeling fragmented and blown about by the experience, they had nothing to grab for stability. Without any such anchor, they became rapidly aware of their inability to move, to act or, in some cases, to even think clearly. The experience of not-knowing was, for this group, profoundly disorienting.

The final embodied description had to do with an awareness of tremendous pressure and crushing weight. This was not solely the abstracted weight of responsibility or pressure to act but more narrowly the *physical* sense of crushing weight. In some cases, this was connected to the abstracted pressures of responsibility, job role, or expected outcomes, but even in these circumstances, the descriptions remained tangible and embodied. Youth workers drew on several vivid images and similes to describe this pressure; all returned to a common thread of being crushed under the pressure of such burdensome weight.

Across all variations, the inability to act remained constant. It struck me (and, in subsequent discussions of the themes with other youth workers in various settings, it struck them, as well) that this inability is different from uncertainty. It is not enough to say that youth workers find themselves uncertain *how* to act in moments of not-knowing. Nor is it sufficient to suggest that youth workers find themselves unable to respond *effectively* in these moments. Although almost certainly true, such statements fail to encompass the desperation evident in this theme. In addition to being uncertain how to act, these variations illustrate youth workers' senses of themselves as fundamentally and almost physically *incapable* of acting—not just effectively, but in any way at all.

In all cases, regardless of its point of origin (isolation, anchorlessness, or pressure), the descriptions of youth workers' inability to act in moments of not-knowing were embodied. This is, first and foremost, a physical reaction. Drizzt described his body this way: "My body was tense. There wasn't much speech . . . just kind of lock-jawed." Along with Ophelia, who said she felt numb throughout the experience, Drizzt described himself as frozen. Lily, extending the bodily reaction somewhat, highlighted her sense of time in relation to her inability to act. She said the experience of not-knowing was "an eternal moment . . . almost like being sucked into a black hole, when you're at the event horizon, when you can't get any closer and you can't get any further away. You're just stuck there. It feels like everything's stuck."

Others described the moment like being under a spotlight or being transfixed by lights. This sense of being "a deer in the headlights," transfixed in spite of the direness of the situation, prevents all further action. It is complete paralysis. Ophelia first used this phrase, and others followed her with the same language. When this happens in phenomenology—when interview participants use the same phrases to describe events that might differ in the nature of the details—it suggests to the analyst that the phrases are nested with meaning beyond the literal. The notion of a deer in the headlights struck me as such a phrase, and it emerged quickly as the core of this theme. It illustrates the heart of the experience in language that makes it both familiar and accessible. On a deeper level, it provides rich soil for interpretation. Like moments of not-knowing, the implications of the metaphor are certainly dire. After all, the deer in the headlight is not only confused and paralyzed, as we often use the phrase to mean. On a deeper level, the deer is also facing a very real danger; if it cannot regroup and move, it may be crushed by the car in whose beams it is transfixed. For many youth workers, the embodied sense of stuckness can feel as dangerous and unsettling as standing in the way of an oncoming car.

It's Just Me and That's Not Enough

Isolation is a dominant feature in the experience of not-knowing. Youth workers are not always alone in moments of not-knowing, although this is often the case. Yet one may feel isolated or alone in the presence of other people. The common feature is the youth worker's sense of disconnection and loss of direction. Regardless of setting or surroundings, the dominant feeling is one of isolation—of being lost. The narratives I heard began with the precursors to the feeling of being lost: heightened energy and confusion followed by the panicked realization that one's own resources or skills are insufficient for the problem at hand. Inadequacy amid isolation—with nowhere to turn for help or guidance—becomes the defining feature of the moment and prevents further action.

Many youth workers likened the experience of isolation to being lost in the wilderness. It is an apt comparison. As with the image of the deer in the headlights, I immediately saw the fit between this metaphor and not-knowing in youth work. Starting in my sixth-grade outdoor school program, I remember learning that, should I become lost in the woods, my immediate response should be to stay put. Moving about, trying to get "unlost" again, is a near-certain recipe for becoming even more lost. I was told to sit still and wait for someone to come help me. Hikers carry whistles for this very purpose; in the event they lose their way, they stop walking and blow their whistles to signal other hikers to their location.

Of course, knowing and doing are different things. In the moment of being lost in the woods, one seldom *actually* thinks rationally about one's actions. I remember, as a young adult, becoming lost on a hike in the mountains of the Pacific Northwest. Rather than calmly reflecting, "I'm lost. I think I'll sit down and wait to be found," my inclination was to panic. My heart raced as I broke out in a cold sweat, and I began to search for the path that I was sure would lead me back to my group. I scrambled to make sense of my surroundings, even while desperately hoping and looking for the arrival of someone else to help me find my way. All the while, I became paralyzed by my own fear, my own sense of isolation and aloneness. The forest became increasingly close, all the bushes began to look similar, and the paths blended together. As I realized that no other hikers were on their way, I fell down, afraid, alone, and unable to act.

Youth workers use similar language to describe their bodily reactions to not-knowing what to do. Echoing the youth worker in the vignette, Stella talked about the heightened energy she experienced as she became conscious of her own isolation. Realizing that she did not know how to respond to the situation her client presented, she began to feel frenetic and scattered. Stella became aware of the "sort of energy where suddenly [everything] is heightened, and you're . . . speaking faster and [with] higher energy and kind of a little bit manic." She associated the experience with that of being suddenly and unexplainably afraid—the kind of fear that prevents action—like being a child in bed who knows a monster lurks in the closet but who cannot call out for help or check the closet for herself. Likewise, in the moment of not-knowing, the scrambling, frenetic energy is present, becoming overpowering and leaving the youth worker both unable to act and unable to call out for help.

Stephanie added to these descriptions, saying that just before realizing she had no resources but her own, everything "feels racy. Like you can hear your blood in your brain." For her, the sense of paralysis described in the first variation came from that raciness. She began to feel too detached to react, divided within herself between the need to seek help and the desire to wait for that help to arrive. It became disorienting: "I'm watching and just seeing [the same thing over and over], and then another part of me that's trying to manage my body, my physical safety... it feels very fragmented." Struggling to pull these threads together and, at the same time, recognizing her inability to move through the fragmented experience, Stephanie reached the height of isolation. Looking around for someone to help, she realized, "Right. It's just me. And that's not enough right now."

This is the moment of being alone in the woods. The heightened energy, the tension between rational and instinctual urges—both reflect the experience of fear that comes from being lost and the uncertainty of how to go about being found again. Stephanie's final reaction, "It's just me, and that's not enough right now," reflects the heavy weight being lost represents for youth workers. We come to our relationships with young people expecting (and being expected) to, at the very least, have some idea of "where we're going and where we have been." This is part of the unspoken therapeutic contract; our role in the relationship is to find and steer a course toward improved outcomes for the youth walking with us. With that understanding, within the contractual and ethical obligation (present, even if implicit) to help, the realization that we ourselves have lost our compass and are lost in the woods is unsettling to the extreme. We may begin to fear not only for ourselves but also for the youth who are trusting us to hold the compass upon which we both rely.

Some youth workers spoke of the sense of paralyzed isolation in a different way. Stephanie and Eve both described panicking at the realization that they were alone and had no way to make meaning of the circumstances they faced. Despite being surrounded by other people, Stephanie was acutely aware of her isolation:

> I'm having a reality that other people are not having. I don't know what the rules are, I don't know how to protect myself, and I'm not seeing anybody else here who's rushing to protect me. I don't know how to respond. I don't understand the context for how other people are responding. Somebody's gonna come help me, right? Nobody did.

Searching for context through the reactions of other people and receiving no feedback in return, Stephanie felt a blend of confusion and paralysis: How could she respond effectively if she could not even understand what had happened? This is echoed in the vignette, as well, in the youth worker's realization that his peers had one another to bounce ideas off, while he had only himself and his own (insufficient) resources.

In many sectors of the field, from group care to street outreach and work in drop-in centers, youth workers function as members of peer units. Outreach is conducted in pairs, at least. Group homes are staffed by rotating teams to ensure that several sets of eyes are always "on." In many cases, youth work is not a solitary activity but one that is informed by and dependent upon active sharing of knowledge and experience. Youth workers are, therefore, often accustomed to working together in teams, using one another as sounding boards and partners, generating intervention strategies through consultation, and often even "tag-teaming" troubling situations. In this light, the recognition that one is alone in an experience—even while surrounded by peers, as was the case for Stephanie—is troubling.

It's Like a Mental Freefall

While for some the sense of paralysis comes from a realization of their isolation, others associate it with a bodily sense of anchorlessness and detachment. In this variation, the inability to respond remains paramount, but its origin is different. Youth workers talked about being unable to act because they were unable to *make* their bodies function properly. Stephanie, who experienced some features of isolation as well as anchorlessness, described feeling out-of-body, as if she had been pulled outside of herself and forced to watch from the outside as she attempted to resolve the issue at hand. Others echoed this image, calling to mind notions of a lack of grounding, anchorlessness, and free-floating weightlessness. The significant feature of this variation is the absolute lack of foundation or direction, without which the youth worker has no basis for action or, even more pointedly, no ability to act.

The image of an anchor ran through several narratives and has emerged as one of the images most resonant with youth workers in my workshops and teaching on the experience of not-knowing. It is a useful image, conveying both stability and freedom. When a boat is anchored or a hot air balloon is tethered, it is secured firmly to the ground. At the same time, however, the boat itself is not grounded, nor is the balloon. One might expect to hear this kind of imagery in a description of not-knowing. I had certainly expected that youth workers would talk about feeling grounded, a term often used in our field to denote a centered, anchored presence. I did not, however, hear that phrase. Instead, youth workers spoke of anchoring—again, nearly across the board, this is the term that emerged. Where *grounding* implies complete immobility (often, as in nautical or disciplinary usage, with a negative connotation), possessing a solid anchor implies that the anchored object has some freedom of mobility but that this mobility is confined within reasonable, predictable, and constant limits. As long as the balloon is tethered to the ground, its pilot knows precisely how high it will float and exactly how to return to the ground should the weather prove unmanageable. The same principle applies for the captain of an anchored ship. Both examples convey stability while allowing for an acceptable and predictable range of motion.

Being anchorless, on the other hand, implies the absolute absence of either grounding or direction. When a ship loses its anchor, it eventually drifts with the current and becomes vulnerable to the direction and force of the sea. As the vignette demonstrates, in moments of not-knowing, paralysis can come directly from being such a ship, anchorless and adrift. In such circumstances, the captain has little more control over the vessel than Stephanie did over her own body; the captain, like her, is left to virtually stand outside, watching the situation from an external vantage point. Without the connection to something constant or stable, such as that provided by an anchor, Stephanie described feeling panicked: "Like I'm just out here, flapping around and I didn't know what to do. It just didn't feel connected [waving her arms around in front of her as though feeling for something in the dark]. Kind of out of body and really pulled out of the situation." The fragmentation of being bodily stuck in the moment and mentally outside of it is profound. As Stephanie's interview gesture implied, it is like hunting in the dark for something you know to be there but cannot see.

For youth workers, accustomed to and expected to provide some direction or foundation to the youth with whom they work, the sense of their own anchorlessness or weightless floating is particularly troublesome. Lacking the connotations of placid calm that might accompany descriptions of weightlessness in other settings, this floating carries a tone of suspension, panic, and an absence of control.

As Lily put it, it is "like a mental freefall. Like you're staring at somebody and your mind is absolutely blank. It's... a kind of disbelief." The experience of the freefall is one, as described by Lily and others, of complete blankness: the awareness of the fall precludes any other thought, engagement, or action. It is this weightlessness, combined with the paralysis of rushing wind that leads to immobility.

Similar to the metaphor of the deer in the headlights, the image of freefalling is apt for its ultimate implications more than its literal description. In this context, weightlessness is profoundly unpleasant. Lily's description, after all, refers to falling from an airplane. She does not refer to the free-floating, cartwheeling weightlessness of astronauts drifting around a space shuttle. Instead, Lily describes a freefall that transfixes motion, leading to a constriction of voluntary mobility: an enforced paralysis. At the same time, taken to its ultimate conclusion, the notion of a freefall is suggestive of the power (potentially deadly) of gravity; the detachment of weightlessness is coupled with impending impact. As with anchorlessness, the sensation is not calming. On the contrary, it is an inability to direct one's own motion in the midst of potentially dangerous outcomes.

The awareness of these outcomes, however vague, is nonetheless present. Adrift in the ocean, the ship captain has some awareness of the severity of the situation. So too does the skydiver. Both are aware of the drift or the rapidly approaching ground. In both cases, there is a sense of looming doom from which there is no clear escape. The same is true for the paralysis of not-knowing. This is a point of connection between this variation and the variation of paralysis-through-isolation; in the moment of mental freefall or the awareness of anchorlessness, the youth worker possesses enough presence of mind to worry about the outcome and long for some way to interrupt it. However, as Sweet Pea put it, "There was no help... just what I had to go by... what I *personally* had to go by." In the midst of the freefall, that's not enough.

That Crushing Becomes Your World

While some experienced the paralysis of not-knowing as weightless or not anchored, for others the paralysis stemmed from a feeling of being held in place or smothered. These narratives described a physical sense of crushing pressure preventing youth workers from responding. This is not only the pressure of responsibility or of perceived expectations, however; such pressure is more reflective and interpretive than what dominated these narratives. The pressure described by Sweet Pea, Lily, Eve, and others was entirely physical and became all-consuming. They described the pressure as confining and constricting in the same way that a straitjacket is constricting; its very purpose is to restrain, to prevent mobility. In this way, the effect of the crushing pressure is similar to that of anchorlessness; both completely prevent action. In both cases, the experience of immobility, rather than its source, becomes the defining characteristic of the moment. We lose our ability to concentrate on the events contributing to our moment of stuckness, focusing all our energy instead on the very fact of that stuckness (which then, of course, contributes to the experience of being stuck).

Contrary to the other variations, in which the youth worker possessed an awareness of both paralysis and potential outcome, narratives highlighting paralysis-through-pressure spoke of the overpowering nature of the pressure itself. In other words, contrary to the mental freefall, where the youth worker is conscious both of the constraints of the fall and the impending impact, those who experienced paralysis resulting from pressure described the moment as myopic. Lily said it felt like "without the pain, the feeling of a migraine. It's like someone taking a big huge pillow and crushing it around your entire head, and leaving this tiny space for you to see out of." The pressure of the pillow prevented her from acting and reduced her awareness to only the tiniest point of focus. Nothing but the pressure remained for her. Lily identified this as the hallmark of her paralysis, when the frustration of not-knowing wrapped so tightly around her that she could see nothing else.

This is, perhaps, one of the defining elements of this variation. Lily and others mentioned that, in the moment, part of the paralysis comes from recognizing that the crushing pressure has edged out all other experiences. Lily said it simply, "That crushing becomes your world." It is as if, in the moment of the worst migraine headache, the rest of the world ceases to exist. All that remains is the pressure, the weight of the moment. As the pressure prevents the youth worker from acting, it also prevents any other perceptions or awareness from entering. It is a self-perpetuating cycle; the more energy that is put toward focusing on the paralysis or the pressure, the more pronounced the pressure becomes. As it becomes more pronounced, more energy is directed toward focusing on it.

Eventually, as Lily described, the crushing becomes your world and even the details that gave rise to it fade from sight. All that is left is the tiny, myopic tunnel vision and a profound and dark sense of weight.

In addition to Lily's description of the inability to focus on anything other than the pressure, Eve and Sweet Pea spoke of pressure in language that called attention to its devastating power. Both structured their narratives around phrases or images that were not only vivid but visceral, possessed of a kind of mortal danger. Eve described the weight of her situation as crushing. Feeling completely insufficient to face the task at hand and aware of the fact that she had no resources but her own from which to draw, she felt at once paralyzed and fragile. She said, "It's like frailty. Y'know, like being crushed by something that's so much bigger [than me] . . . it's just kind of getting crushed by that." There is, in this description, a sense of desperation born from the fear of obliteration. It is as if, unable to focus on anything other than this pressure, Eve feared the loss of herself—being crushed by and disappearing beneath the weight of that pressure.

In something of a contrast to some of the other participants, Sweet Pea described her experience similarly but emphasized the weight of her own paralysis combined with the fear of what might come if she remained in a place of not-knowing (similar to what others experienced with references to free-falling or feeling like deer in the headlights). She described feeling frozen under the pressure of not-knowing: "It was horrible. Just a lot of pressure. Like everything that's about to happen weighs on me. Just so heavy on my shoulders." In this way, the pressure of not-knowing becomes blended with other pressures: the pressure to act, the pressure to solve, the pressure to perform. As with Eve, the unspoken fear comes through: what if I fail to withstand this pressure? Pressure blends with expectation and vocational or professional obligation in a way that effectively guarantees immobility.

Chapter 6

Helpless, Hopeless, and Out of Control: Features of Despair

SUMMARY. Youth workers often pride themselves on the degree to which they share power with clients, encounter clients on their own terms, and allow young people to set the tone for and direct the helping relationship. In their descriptions of not-knowing, however, many youth workers mention acute discomfort at the feeling of control having been stripped away from them rather than willingly surrendered or shared. This chapter describes the second of five themes associated with youth workers' experiences of not knowing what to do: the loss of control and features of despair. In addition to presenting the dominant theme of helplessness and loss of control, this chapter discusses the three variations on the theme, as described by youth worker participants: (a) There was nothing there to protect me, (b) Something else just took control of everything, and (c) What does he have to do, kill someone?!

VIGNETTE: LISA, WHY WON'T YOU HELP US?

My most conscious moment of not-knowing came when I had been working with Justin's family for about 3 months. Justin was a tough kid, there's no doubt about it. He was about 10 or 11 and, at the time of this team meeting, he had just been expelled from school for saying he was going to bring an Uzi to school and kill all his teachers. Already on probation, he now faced a felony charge for terroristic threats. Things were getting serious.

They were serious at home, too. He had become so frightening to his parents—threatening to boil the family cat, throwing himself through locked windows when sent to his room, cursing family members in the most vulgar language they had ever heard, and more—that his father had recently quit his job just so they could both be home with him. Justin's dad was about to be shipped overseas (he was in the Army Reserves), and nobody knew what to do. His parents were desperate, the state social worker wanted him removed from the home but couldn't find reasonable cause in the eyes of the court, and the probation officer had no recourse because juvenile detention refused to take such a young child. On paper, I was supposed to be the counselor, the representative of the mental health system. In reality, it felt more like I was supposed to fix this kid.

But I didn't know how to fix him. I didn't know how to do anything helpful for anyone involved. We were all desperate, and we were getting more and more frustrated as time went on. I remember I tried all these different interventions—everything I could think of to help this family—but Justin just kept getting worse. It's not like he was just *getting* worse; it's like he was *choosing* to be worse. Every time we'd try something, he would up the ante. There was so much energy around trying to figure out what was wrong with him, why he was acting the way he acted, and what we could do about it. I can't ever remember working so hard on one case . . . but nothing ever seemed to be any better. In fact, it just kept getting worse.

Working with this kid was like a tornado: Everything kept spiraling out of control, whipping everything around him into a frenzy! His behavior scared his parents more and more. He was causing damage all over their house, breaking windows, destroying walls. I would suggest an intervention, and then he'd jump right over the top of it. There was no containing him, no controlling anything. I remember just feeling completely out of control, like watching a storm approach but not being able to get out of its way. I knew I was also getting sucked into that storm, and there was nothing I could do to avoid it. I didn't know what to do. It was everything I could do to just keep my feet on the ground. Everything felt like it was just moving so fast—I couldn't regain control over anything—I was just responding to this, and then responding to that, and I never knew really where anything was headed. It was just react, react, react! Dodge, dodge, dodge! What wall are we going to hit with this kid? How bad do things have to get? When is this going to stop?!

And then, at this team meeting, I was sitting in a room with Justin's mom and dad. They were looking at me with their eyes all sunk down in their heads. They looked terrible, completely exhausted and worn. They seemed so sad. His mom looked up at me with tears in her eyes and asked, "Lisa, why won't you *help* us?" I had no idea what to say. I couldn't respond. I *wanted* to help them, but I didn't know what else to *do*.

I could feel my defenses just crumbling around me. I'm supposed to be a professional, right? I'm supposed to be able to maintain some kind of emotional distance between me and my clients. But this situation just cut right through all that. Seeing Justin's mom in tears, knowing the pain *he* must be going through in order to keep behaving like this, and being totally unable to do anything about it—it just cut right through everything I had. There was nothing left to shield me, to protect me from their pain, their fear, their frustration. I tried to hang on to my professionalism, but it was crumbling. It's like I was grasping at the edge of a cliff, but the dirt was falling through my fingers. My heart was pounding. My mind was racing, trying to think of *something* helpful to say. But there just wasn't anything. Just her voice, "Why won't you *help* us?" I felt so useless, so helpless.

I felt so frustrated, just being stuck in that moment, without any sense of what I could or should do to help this kid, this family. There was so much wrong with the situation! He was too young for juvi (juvenile detention), his parents were too dedicated to him for him to be in foster care, he showed too much deliberate control over his actions to be called psychotic and hospitalized. There was nothing to do. I mean, socially, there was nothing. There were no real resources for this family. Why won't I help them? Because I can't. There's nothing I can do. I wanted to stand up and scream, at the top of my lungs, "It's not fair!!!" But that's not good enough. That's not a very good answer. That's just the way the world is, and there's no resolution right now. I was just so sad about that, about not knowing what to do about that, how to fight it.

Having to tell them that was so hard. It's like being with someone dealing with death. There's nothing you can do to make their grief go away. You don't know how to make it better. You just don't know how, and there's probably not anything you *can* do, anyway. You just have to sit with it. I just had to sit with things the way they were. It's a hopeless situation, when you just have to figure out how to keep going, without any real hope that things are going to be any different tomorrow. I didn't know what else to do. I just didn't know.

HELPLESS, HOPELESS, AND OUT OF CONTROL

Where the previous theme (like a deer in the headlights) dealt with youth workers' physical paralysis in moments of not-knowing, this theme is organized around the despair and futility associated with not knowing what to do in a situation where a response is imperative. Almost without exception, the youth workers in the study commented that their profound sadness during and after the moment of not-knowing was a reaction they felt a professional obligation not to share, even with colleagues and supervisors. Their stories of not-knowing were most often shared, if at all, in the context of trading war stories or supplying comic relief in social encounters; naming the despair and futility included in them felt to these workers like a transgression of some implied youth worker code. This enforced silence contributed an additional layer of sadness to their experience of not-knowing.

Despair of this sort is difficult to manage, largely because it strikes a personal, emotional cord. With regard to their experiences of not-knowing, youth workers who participated in the study talked about the despair and futility associated with losing control and about questions associated with the value of their work. This was not the vocational question about the utility of youth work generally. On the contrary, workers described deeply personal experiences of feeling out of control, helpless, exposed, and despondent as the result of their inability to respond to a situation. These were not fleeting reactions. In fact, one of the central features of the variation is its duration. This is not the immediate recognition of paralysis, as in the previous variation. Instead, it is the apprehensive sense of impending loss of control mixed with the long-term emotional pain of having been unable to help.

Three significant variations on this theme emerged from the interviews and have been supported by other youth workers in workshops and classes subsequent to this study. First, most youth workers experienced futility as preceded by an awareness of the wearing down of their defenses. They described not-knowing as an eroding force, slowly crumbling the defenses they had been professionally trained to maintain. With no psychic or emotional defenses left to buffer them from the experiences of their clients (or the frustration and pain of those experiences), youth workers described feeling helpless and even childlike.

Others experienced the despair and futility of not-knowing through the image of control. Youth workers in this group described their conscious awareness of a moment during which the energy in the encounter became exaggerated, like the tornado in the vignette that opened this chapter. In these cases, youth workers found themselves gradually (in some cases rapidly) losing control of themselves, of their decision-making abilities, and of the situation in general. Feeling uncomfortable, even panicked, they desperately scrambled to regain control and maintain some veneer of professional calm and demeanor. At the height of not-knowing, they became aware that they could not maintain this image, that they may be letting other people down as a result, and that there was little else they could do. Still in the midst of the tornado, youth workers in this group had no way out of the storm. Worse, they were convinced beyond doubt that the storm was partially of their creation and that they, like their clients, were likely to be hurt (emotionally and possibly professionally) in the destruction it left in its path. This loss of control of self and situation left these workers with a deep sense of sadness and futility.

The final variation, closely linked to the futility of being out of control, related directly to the sense of hopelessness youth workers experienced upon encountering situations too large for them to resolve. This is not only about the situations themselves, however. It is more precisely connected to the youth workers' inability to respond to them. For instance, watching clients experience the abuses of racism or responding to the social service delivery system's inability to provide much-needed intervention and respite wore down the youth workers' faith in their ability to do their jobs. Voicing this doubt, Athena wondered at how to keep going in the midst of "not knowing what to do about that [racism], not knowing how to change it, not knowing how to fight that, not knowing how to make amends for that situation." There is a palpable feeling of hopelessness in her experience, a hopelessness born out of the a larger sense of social futility characterized by the realization that she and her client were, together, up against something far too large for either of them to impact.

It struck me, in discussing this theme with other youth workers, that its variations are related to one another in a different way than in other themes. For instance, although youth workers who experience being stuck in the moment of not-knowing may identify some combination of the variations (like Lily, who described both feeling out-of-body and feeling very stuck in her body at different times in the experience), each variation is distinct. In describing their experiences of futility and despair, however, many youth workers presented the variations in a circular fashion. That is, many participants spoke of a realization that their defenses were crumbling, which contributed to the feeling of losing control, which then bled into hopelessness and despair. With the realization that their personal and professional protections were melting away, they began to feel out of control and helpless. Similar to the crushing pressure described in the previous theme, this helplessness soon dominated their awareness. Having lost their defenses contributed to their sense that the entire situation was spiraling out of control. From this point, it was only a short step to the realization of their own futility and possibly even the futility of their efforts, which introduced deep despair against which they had no remaining defenses.

There Was Nothing There to Protect Me

As the previous theme illustrated, one of the hallmarks of not-knowing is its overwhelming magnitude. Vanessa spoke clearly of feeling threatened, seeking to escape the frustration of not-knowing before it became too overwhelming. There is a sense of danger associated with being overwhelmed, a potential to be lost beneath the weight of whatever comes. After all, in order for something to be overwhelming, there must be something else (something smaller, weaker) to be overwhelmed. Youth workers identified themselves as those smaller, weaker, potentially overwhelmed "somethings" attempting to protect themselves from drowning in the emotional difficulty of their work. This is common among the helping professions; helpers must find ways of keeping themselves separate from and outside of the pain or confusion their clients experience. We structure countless hours of professional and academic training, in-service, and supervision around the development and maintenance of boundaries and self-care strategies for just this reason. At times, however, those protections fail, as often happens in moments of not-knowing.

This failure of the defenses is central to many people's experiences of not-knowing. At the height of the moment, the uncertainty, pressure, and despair of not-knowing overwhelm the youth worker's protections. It is a graphic and violent image: The threatening presence of the weight of not-knowing looming over the defensive walls of the youth worker's sense of self, professionalism, and obligation to her clients. For many, as this dangerous sense of fear, frustration, and doom grows, the urgency to respond and the parallel inability to react intensify. As their defenses break down, youth workers feel increasingly vulnerable to the panicked and overwhelmed despair of not-knowing.

Eve described the crumbling of her defenses in very vivid language. Using militaristic imagery, she talked about not-knowing as though she were describing a city under siege. Under attack from the pressure of the event, she found herself scrambling to maintain the boundaries and internal defenses that enabled her to continue doing her job in spite of the overwhelming confusion of not-knowing. Having been trained in the professional attached detachment of boundaries in residential care work, of Eve felt safe having "all these walls up to protect me," until the moment of not-knowing. As the moment wore on, she identified an acute "sense of being so attacked and feeling so vulnerable . . . just having the defenses broken down bit by bit. They're just crumbling. There was nothing to protect me from anything."

She went on to talk about her awareness of these defenses crumbling. It was a descriptor she used often. Intrigued by her use of crumbling, (partially since other participants had used the same term in describing this experience), I asked Eve what that was like. She immediately replied with metaphors like "standing on a very small island as the surf crumbles away the shoreline" or "clinging by my fingers to a cliffside and having the ground crumble under my fingers." Similarly, Stella described the experience as one of vulnerability, watching as her defenses melted around her, almost as if they were wax objects before a fire.

These images, melting and crumbling, convey profound meanings. Embedded in the idea of crumbling is an acute awareness of time. Crumbling and melting differ, after all, from snapping or breaking. The experience Eve and Stella described is slow. It is not a sudden failure of their defenses, not water bursting through a hole in the dam, but rather a slow, gradual falling apart. Crumbling takes time. It is a process one watches, not a split-second occurrence that happens quickly and is over. Helpless to do anything else, stuck youth workers must watch as their defenses crumble, an image that calls to mind the interminable moment of impending doom. Watching a cliff crumble or a wave crash on a sand castle, one knows the ultimate outcome: The cliffside will fall, and the castle will wash away. Crumbling is the gradual state of not-quite-but-soon-to-be-fallen. In this context, watching the defenses crumble suggests that the youth worker knows the doom that is coming and must wait for that outcome to arrive. There is little to be done other than watch and wait.

The heightened sense of impending doom is strengthened by youth workers' descriptions of *what* is crumbling. They invoked military language that conjured up violent and dangerous images. They spoke of defenses, walls, and protections, none of which is a valueless term. On the contrary, each presumes something specific: An attack from which one must be defended, sheltered, or protected. It is like standing on the walls of a besieged city, watching the invading army amass on the plain outside. One knows that, sooner or later, the walls will be breached. Sooner or later, the war will be lost. Watching their defenses crumble, youth workers' sense of that doom, the urgency of the moment, is heightened. After all, in Eve's imagery, what will come of her when the island is submerged or the cliff gives way completely? For many youth workers, the answer is frightening to the point of paralysis.

Ophelia talked about the meaning of watching her defenses crumble. She began by talking about how she prepared herself for her work. To keep herself from personalizing painful or difficult situations in her interactions with youth, she said, "I zip myself up and I have a protective barrier around myself. I envision something that's protecting me." In the moment of not-knowing, "That was sort of crumbling. That wasn't there anymore." Without those defenses in place, she felt shaken and vulnerable. Although she wanted to be strong and in control, present to help support the young person and his family, the realization that her defenses had crumbled made her feel "pretty whimpery. Just not strong. Not like an adult. Sort of like a child." Feeling small and out of control, she was vulnerable to all the turmoil and confusion of the situation. As her defenses crumbled, the waves came crashing through, threatening to drown Ophelia beneath them.

For Ophelia, in addition to being unpleasant, this was also a breach of the implied contract between her (as a youth worker) and her client. Like many of her peers, Ophelia operated under an assumption that she must maintain a sense of professionalism or emotional detachment (although youth work, more than other fields, certainly encourages us to blend our personal or emotional selves with our professional roles). This emotional detachment allows youth workers to convey an image of stability while also protecting themselves from the psychic toll of youth work. In this way, maintaining a professional image of poise and confidence is not merely desirable. In fact, we tell ourselves that it is essential, that parents and youth rely on the stability and confidence our professional faces convey. It is crucial for ourselves, as well, since we often use this professional façade as a line of defense, enabling us to expose ourselves to emotionally exhausting and traumatic experiences without suffocating beneath them.

So what happens when that veneer crumbles? It, like our other defenses, can melt in the heat of not-knowing. Drizzt's experience, mirroring Lisa's in the vignette, highlights the despair that accompanies the youth worker's realization that his or her professional image has been compromised, that even that most basic defense has been eroded. It is a desperate position, attempting to manage the fear and doom of one's own defenses crumbling while also maintaining the professional face one believes the client needs to see. Feeling the futility that comes with melting protections, Drizzt said, "Being caught between keeping a professional face and being in that [desperate] space . . . you've gotta keep going. But it's hard. It's tiring." The tension between these positions, the personal and the professional, is exhausting. It is also seldom discussed.

Something Else Just Took Control of Everything

For some youth workers, losing control is the direct result of crumbled defenses. In this way, it is an extension of the previous variation rather than a distinct variation itself. For others, however, it is a discrete experience. Losing control is central to the experience of not-knowing for this group. Involving both personal and professional implications (losing control over oneself as well as over the situation in general), the act of losing control was central for many of the study's participants. They described how becoming aware of the loss of control (or of losing control) introduced heightened sensitivity to their bodies, their sense of relationship and space, and their ability to maintain a detached and professional demeanor. Many youth workers used graphic and vivid imagery to describe not only the experience of losing control but also the fear and desperation wrapped up in that experience.

Control represents an interesting tension for youth workers. We are trained to see ourselves as partners with youth and to applaud ourselves for letting go of the need to control or direct the situations or circumstances our clients present. In fact, this positioning ourselves as aligned with youth, rather than above them (as is the often unintended consequence of an intervention or problem-solving stance), has emerged as a hallmark of American youth work. It has become a standard around which youth workers can rally and stake their unique contribution or role among the helping professions. We resist interventions that place the onus of control upon us, preferring instead to bolster and celebrate our clients' abilities to control their own lives. At the same time, however, we expect ourselves to possess some measure of control over our own behaviors, thoughts, and interventions. Although we partner with youth, we are not *merely* their partners; we are also their helpers, their teachers, their guides. In order to help, we must have some indication of where we are headed, what to do next, and how to go about that process.

What happens, then, when we lose control? There is richness in that phrase. After all, losing control is different from giving it up. As previously mentioned, youth workers tend to be fairly comfortable voluntarily giving up control. When we "meet youth where they're at," we say we have given control over to young people to direct their own lives. Losing control, however, conjures up a completely different emotional reaction. The loss of control implies having been in control at one point; one cannot lose something one never possessed. It is also involuntary, forced, and uncomfortable. We notice things we have lost only when we miss their presence, and if they hold value for us, we often go to great lengths to recover them. The same is true in the field; we are comfortable operating with our clients in control *except* when we have not voluntarily given over that control.

The despair and futility associated with the experience of not-knowing relates directly, for many youth workers, to precisely this experience of losing control. Unlike some other variations, it is an experience youth workers have no difficulty describing. For instance, Eve talked about her loss of control in urgent and physical language. Watching her defenses crumble and recognizing that she was about to lose control, she described leaving her body. As her energy heightened, she lost touch with her rational self. She said, "My sense of myself just totally disappeared into this completely instinctual place where the only thing that mattered was making it stop." She had no resources, though, for making [the moment of stuckness] stop. Being so out of control, she felt like she had blacked out, like "[her] body took [her] somewhere else" and she didn't return until the moment had passed. For Eve, it was simply impossible to continue upon realizing she had lost control. Hers was a visceral experience resulting from and exaggerating her sense of defenseless vulnerability in the face of not-knowing.

Drizzt, too, described the loss of control in physical terms, but for him it was not connected to the experience of crumbling defenses. Nevertheless, in the height of not-knowing, he found himself caught in the frantic energy and quickened pace of the situation spiraling out of his control. In language similar to Lisa's in the vignette, Drizzt described feeling frantic and pressured. He likened the experience to being in but not steering a speeding car. Wheels spinning out of control, the situation was "flying fast, like we ain't got no brakes. Man! Where's this gonna stop? We need it to stop! It's just, 'buzzzzzzz!' What are we gonna hit?! We've got to slow down!" Completely out of control, Drizzt was unable to get out of the car; he was paralyzed in the moment of not-knowing, conscious only of his own inability to control or influence the situation and the ultimate outcome of the impending crash. In this case, the experience was precisely related to the futility of his role. With no shred of control over the situation, Drizzt became consumed by the apprehension and fear that came from the recognition of his own helplessness.

In both cases, the experience of losing control was not limited simply to the act of being out of control. As Drizzt illustrated, it also included a clear sense of something even worse to come, something the youth worker can see but cannot prevent. This awareness—that a crash is imminent—is similar to the experience of watching one's defenses crumble. It also illustrates not-knowing's pervasive feature of looming disaster in a way that mirrors the previous experience of being stuck like a deer in the headlights. It is characterized by desperation, a panicked longing for the experience to end in spite of the youth worker's inability to stop it. Further, these narratives demonstrate that although they, themselves, have no control over the situation at the height of not-knowing, youth workers possess an awareness that they (as much as their clients) will be involved in whatever negative outcomes ensue. Drizzt's entire narrative is phrased in the plural: "*We* ain't got no brakes . . . what are *we* gonna hit?!" It is a heavy and desperate weight to carry, being implicated in the disaster over which you have no control and which you are powerless to prevent. Knowing this but not knowing what to do about it (or being able to do anything even if a course of action were to be seen) becomes overwhelming. After all, in such a situation, the youth worker's ethical obligation kicks in: he cannot merely call an end to the session and send the client home to manage this frustration alone. Everyone shares in the consequences of the youth worker's loss of control.

What Does He Have to Do, Kill Someone?

The despair of not-knowing is not solely related to the crumbling of defenses or the loss of control. In many cases, youth workers identified the moment as forcing them to come to terms with their own potential uselessness. Haunted by their inability to surmount the barriers presented to their clients, whether these are due to the sudden death of a close friend, exposure to social inequities like racism, or the limitations of the social service network, youth workers find themselves hopelessly questioning their usefulness. This is not the question of whether youth work itself is worthwhile; that is a deeper vocational question that did not arise during these interviews. Instead, this sense of uselessness, highlighting the futility of one's position in a given moment, relates directly to the youth worker and the moment. It is a question of *their own* value in this interaction, not about the value of the work itself. On a deeper level, it is a question about the role of hope and hopelessness for the youth worker, of how to keep going in the face of seemingly insurmountable odds and one's own despair at not knowing how to manage. Where other variations concerned the loss of control or breakdown of defenses, this concerns the erosion of hope.

Lori called attention to these questions in relating her experience with youth at a drop-in center after hearing that one of their friends had recently died in a far-away city. Witnessing their pain and having no idea how to respond to it, no ability to make the situation better for any of them, heightened her own grief. Unable to help, not because there was nothing to be done but instead because she did not know what to do, she questioned her own usefulness. The situation began to feel hopeless as she struggled with her value in the moment: "[It]gets to the point where you just get really frustrated, because... you know that you're somewhat useless in this situation... it's beyond your control." This is different from simply working within a resolutionless situation. After all, even hopeless situations can harbor moments of clarity and action. Instead, it is working within that situation while having no idea *how* to be helpful. Paralyzed in the moment of not-knowing, having lost hope in her ability to bring her clients to a better emotional place, Lori started to question her skills as a youth worker: If I truly am useless, as I seem to be, then why am I still here?

Athena, Ophelia, and Vanessa experienced this futile hopelessness differently. In each case, the moment of not-knowing became exaggerated by the recognition that some large-scale and intangible social barrier had closed off their ability to act. Athena, a White woman, described being with a Black client and observing a patently racist interaction in which her client was both silenced and threatened by an older White woman. Her experience of the moment was one of utter hopelessness; Athena not only had no idea how to respond, she also had no hope that her response would actually result in an improved outcome. She became paralyzed in the face of trying to respond in a way that would undo the damage and pain inflicted by racism. She said,

> What do you do when people that you really care about are constantly confronted by racism and there's not a very good answer? That's just the way the world is, and there's no resolution right now. I was just feeling sad about that.

"Just feeling sad" struck me as an understatement when I heard Athena say this. Her sadness, even during our conversation months after the event, brought her to tears. The futility expressed in these statements echoes that of other youth workers who find themselves in situations where macrolevel forces prevent their protection and intervention on behalf of their clients. It is a paralyzing futility born of not knowing how to respond.

Ophelia and Vanessa described similar experiences, commenting on the emotional toll this hopelessness takes on them as fellow human beings, not merely as professionals. Ophelia returned throughout her interview to a sense of profound grief, not merely about her inability to respond but also about the implications of that inability. Recognizing that she had no control over the situation and no defenses left to prepare her for the moment of not knowing what to do, Ophelia worried that her indecision would result in a series of negative outcomes for her client.

This worry, she said, is overwhelming. It, in itself, becomes paralyzing because there is no way to see through the veil it casts over the situation. She said, "It's hopeless. It's sort of like grief. Like when someone dies and you just try to figure out how to still live [her voice trembles as she pats her chest over her heart]. Y'know? That's kind of how it felt." Vanessa used a similar image, suggesting that working within the moment of not-knowing is like working with someone else's grief; there really is nothing you can do to make it go away but neither can you leave the situation. She said, "It's the feeling of not knowing what to say or what to do to make things better but having to sit with things the way they are." Like Lori's, these descriptions illustrate that not-knowing can be a helpless, hopeless experience.

It is an experience that does not end when the encounter is over, either. Invoking the imagery of working through the grief of someone's death, Ophelia's description hints at the long-term effects of this despair. Echoing Lisa's experience from the vignette, Drizzt described the haunting impacts of having been useless precisely because of not knowing what to do. When the mother of a client looked at him, pleading for help that he could not offer, Drizzt felt totally torn and useless. The mother asked, over and over, what her son had to do in order for Drizzt to help—Did he have to kill someone? Remembering the hopelessness of the situation, he said,

> Mom was just [gestures a series of urgent yanks on his shirtsleeves] . . . it was his mom. Just tugging. I had . . . kind of an echo in my ear: "he's [her son] gonna kill somebody, kill somebody, kill somebody . . . " [looks away and laughs as though nervous]. That was haunting me for months.

The awful futility of the realization that his client would possibly need to do something so horrible in order to get the services he obviously needed brought Drizzt to a definite and, in his words, haunting sense of despair and hopelessness for himself, for his client, and for the structures that prevented him from helping this family.

For Drizzt, the height of despair came in his experience of not knowing how to access the services his client so desperately needed. For Athena, it was the result of her encounter with racism. What remains constant across these experiences is the general sense of hopelessness and futility or despair that comes from not-knowing, from having lost control, or from watching, helpless, as one's professional defenses crumble.

Chapter 7

Center Stage: Humiliation, Being Found Out, and the Myth of Supercompetence

SUMMARY. Youth workers operate within a professional climate in which competence is perceived to be linked to a worker's ability to respond quickly and effectively to whatever situations clients may present. Many youth workers perceive their own inability to respond in moments of stuckness as indicative of their own failing and lack of professional skill. They often view their colleagues as more equipped and competent than themselves and fear having their own struggles exposed. This chapter describes the third of five themes associated with youth workers' experiences of not-knowing what to do: humiliation and the fear of being found out. In addition to presenting the dominant theme, this chapter discusses the two variations on the theme, as described by youth worker participants: (a) The worst public humiliation and (b) They'll know I'm a fraud. Implicit in both variations is the weight of youth workers' attempts to measure up to the field's myth of supercompetence in their practice.

VIGNETTE: DRUNK AND DISORDERLY

I was so excited about this conference! Together with the kids we served, my program had raised enough money to bring three youth representatives to a national youth development convention held in New York. Our program was even being featured in one of the breakout sessions. The whole event was a very big production for the agency, a feather in everyone's cap. The staff had spent a lot of time determining which youth to bring, who would best represent the program, and which staff to send. I was excited to be going, a little nervous about being responsible for the youth, and eager to prove myself to the other convention participants.

Still, it was a frightening experience. I had never even been to a national conference before, let alone been responsible for youth at one. I was basically on my own to represent myself, the program, and my agency. The only other person attending from my agency was the executive director, a woman I was desperate to impress. People would be coming to this conference from all over the country, and I was very aware that my work was going to be on display, not only because of the program, but also because I was bringing youth representatives. It was nerve-wracking; I didn't feel quite prepared for that level of publicity.

On the first day of the conference, I remember sitting in the lobby of the hotel, chatting with a large group of staff and directors from other agencies. The lobby was crowded, with small groups of adults and youth everywhere, all waiting for the dining room to open. Mid-sentence, I became distracted by loud noise—yelling and carrying on—coming from somewhere near the front doors. Two youth came stumbling into the lobby, shouting and hooting at the top of their lungs. One was Devin, a youth from my program. They were obviously drunk, as Devin shouted across the room to me, "Yo, Chris! Whassup? How YOU doin'?!"

Hundreds of eyes landed on me at once. Their weight was crushing. Mortified, I started sweating. Totally shaken and completely at a loss for a response, I tried to mumble an excuse to the folks in my group and walked over to Devin. Everyone in the lobby had turned to face us as Devin continued his loud, drunken rambling. I had no idea how to deal with this situation; it just hadn't occurred to me that something like this could happen. I didn't know how to manage the fact that it was happening so publicly. I wanted to grab him and run away to some corner of the hotel and find out what was going on. But I couldn't. For some reason, I couldn't seem to move.

Trying to talk to Devin, I found myself getting very red-faced. I knew all eyes in the lobby were on me, on us, as much to see my response as out of surprise and irritation at his behavior. I started running madly through all the interventions in my mental toolbox, every youth development–appropriate technique I could think of, knowing everyone was watching to see how I was going to handle this. And I found myself unable to do much of anything. I just didn't know what to do. It was like being on stage, opening night, and forgetting your lines—there's nothing you can do. All the next lines are dependent on yours, but you have drawn a blank. Center stage, I was completely exposed, totally out in the open. I could hear people whispering all around the lobby—whispers that echoed through the room. I knew they were whispering about *me*, about what I should do, about how I never should have left Devin, how I *must* be young and brand-new.

Hearing the whispers, frantically trying to figure out what to do next, I was aware of my throat tightening, my chest feeling really tight. The whole hotel suddenly warmed by about 15 degrees. It felt like a huge spotlight was shining right down on this situation, on me, and there was no place I could go to get out of the light. The vulnerability, the exposure, was just about the worst public humiliation I had ever experienced.

It wasn't just that I was embarrassed about Devin, though. It was more that I knew all these people were watching me fumble around not knowing how to respond to him. *They* would know what to do; I was sure of it. My uncertainty was more conspicuous than Devin's drunkenness. I just fumbled about, with no direction or apparent effect. Frantic thoughts kept going through my mind about how I *should* be taking charge, getting all authoritative and directing the show. But for some reason, I couldn't translate any of those thoughts into action. I was just so embarrassed, so shown up. And everyone knew it. All the people I had been chatting with knew that I didn't know how to do my job. Soon, my executive director would know it, too. I wanted to run and hide—but there was nowhere to go. My ineptitude was completely on display. It had become the main attraction.

That was maybe the worst part. The embarrassment was bad enough, but it was even worse to know that I was so ashamed *because* I was inept. Not because Devin had done something stupid, but because *I* didn't know what to do about it. *I* brought him to the conference, after all. I should have known how to deal with whatever might have come up! But I didn't. I felt like such a sham, like this experience was going to expose me to everyone as a total fraud. The whole situation just reinforced my greatest fear: that I go around all the time pretending that I know what I'm doing, but I don't really know anything at all. All these people were going to find out that I don't know anything, really—they're going to see me as a fraud. And then what? What would happen when I had to face my executive director? My supervisor? When other kids in the program back home heard about this? I had been called out as a fraud, and it was going to cost me—almost definitely my job and probably my career. No one wants to hire a fraud.

CENTER STAGE

For many youth workers, the experience of not-knowing brought with it a powerful feeling of embarrassment and shame. Although it contained some physical descriptions, this theme more directly concerned youth workers' assumptions about other people's perceptions of and reactions to them vis-à-vis the situation. That is, in describing the humiliation involved in not-knowing, youth workers consistently talked about their fears of what other people were thinking, their embarrassment about other people finding out they had lost control, or their shame at being found to be a fraud. In the back of their heads throughout the experience of not-knowing, participants remained concerned about how they would be perceived in light of their inability to react.

Two features framed the descriptions of this element of not-knowing. The first involved the publicity of the event. Even in circumstances where they were alone with a client at the moment of not-knowing, as was the case with another worker, Vanessa, participants nonetheless identified a fear of what would happen when their failure became evident. What would her colleagues say *when* (not *if*) they found out she did not know what to do? It was, for most participants, a foregone conclusion that their not-knowing would become public knowledge. For those whose experience occurred in a public setting (like Athena or Cleve), the shame of knowing other people were witness to their inability to act bordered on crippling.

The second feature of these descriptions of humiliation related to error, to participants' sense of having done something wrong—or, more accurately, having failed to do something right. After all, we only become embarrassed about mistakes we believe we should not have committed. Embarrassment and humiliation come from the combined recognition that we have made a mistake and that it could have (and probably should have) been prevented. Youth workers interpreted their moments of not-knowing similarly: they were humiliating precisely because, in their minds, anyone else would have known what to do to prevent or avoid the situation.

This belief, disturbingly pervasive among the youth workers in the study and others across the field (indeed, possibly among the helping professions in general), speaks to what I have come to call the myth of supercompetence. It is the individual belief (often held strongly enough to be a conviction) that I, as a youth worker, should be not only competent but supercompetent in my work. Although our professional rhetoric suggests that no one can expect perfection in practice, since we seldom—if ever—hear one another's not-knowing stories in supervision or even idle conversation with other youth workers, we can allow ourselves to see our colleagues as fundamentally more competent than we are. It is irrational, of course. In moments of clarity, we can see the man behind the curtain and know both that others experience not-knowing and uncertainty, as well, and that our peers are just as normal and human as we are. But in the moment of not-knowing and in managing the humiliation and shame in its wake, youth workers often punish themselves for their inability to perform as supercompetently as they believe they should and as they assume their idealized colleagues would have performed.

These features, publicity and error, framed both of this theme's two variations. The first concerns participants' descriptions of humiliation itself. Youth workers talked specifically about the experience and meaning of the embarrassment they felt in and after the moment of not-knowing. Not only providing rich narrative descriptions of what this public shame felt like, they also offered useful insights into its origins. As previously suggested, the humiliation of not-knowing came, at least in part, from perceived failure on the part of the youth worker, the publicity of the event, and the feeling that the youth worker, due to his or her own failing, had let other people down.

The second variation illustrates how youth workers understood the humiliation of not-knowing. Across the board, they talked about their moment of inability or uncertainty as reflective of the fact that they have no idea how to do their work. Not only should the mistake of not-knowing have been prevented, it is something that *would* have been prevented if the participants had only known what they were doing. The fact that they did not know what to do was interpreted by the youth workers themselves as evidence that they were mere frauds. After all, had they been true professionals, they would have known how to respond. Where this became troubling for the participants is not in the realization that they saw themselves to be, in Cleve's words, "shams." On the contrary, they all accepted that as a given. What was problematic for these youth workers was the fear that their hoax (masquerading as competent professionals while believing themselves to be frauds) was about to be exposed. The public announcement of their incompetence dominated the experience, much more than the uncertainty itself. They felt ashamed because, thanks to the public nature of the situation, everyone (including clients, professional colleagues, and others) *knew* them to be frauds. The experience of not-knowing served as a public confirmation of something the youth workers themselves already believed to be true.

The implications for the field, possibly for the future of American youth work, are clear. No one can avoid moments of not-knowing altogether; to do so requires an impossible omnipotence. As long as individual youth workers hold themselves to this supercompetent standard in a culture of silent shame around their moments of not-knowing, however, they continue to practice under a fear—or a fundamental belief—that they are charlatans. This creates a burden for helpers that is simply too heavy to carry for long. Herein lies the crux of the relationship between not-knowing and burnout. Until youth work, as a field, begins to debunk this myth of supercompetence, individual youth workers, many of whom are extraordinarily skilled in their craft, will continue to leave the field prematurely, demoralized and weary.

THE WORST PUBLIC HUMILIATION

Listening to youth workers talk about the embarrassment and humiliation they experienced as accompanying the moment of not-knowing, I returned again and again to the image of an actor who has forgotten his lines on opening night. The image applies for a number of reasons. First, like actors, youth workers often operate as though independent of their audiences, while being at once acutely aware that their efforts are on display. On stage in the middle of a performance, actors look out into darkness. Although aware of the audience's presence, the actor cannot actually see into the theater. I remember the feeling of being on stage in a production and allowing myself to believe that the room was empty save for my fellow actors on the stage. The blinding lights in my face acted as a screen to protect me from having to face the audience, my critics.

At the same time, of course, actors are sharply aware that the same lights hiding the audience from sight illuminate every one of their own steps and missteps. It creates a baffling sense of isolation and exposure, which echoed participants' sense of being watched even when the moment of not-knowing occurred in the private setting of a counseling session or consultation room. Actors know that, despite the sense of their own private world on the stage, there is actually nowhere under the lights that escapes the notice of those in the audience. In the moment of not-knowing, youth workers described a similar sense of the inevitability that their errors would be put on public display, even when the actual circumstances of the event—when examined rationally—would suggest otherwise. This is the public element of not-knowing, the exposure we fear when we operate within the myth of supercompetence. It is the feature that contributes most directly and heavily to the embarrassment participants described; after all, we only feel embarrassed when we are found out. Our own private failures may be upsetting, but they are only *embarrassing* when they are brought to light.

Returning to the image of the stage, it is one thing for an actor to forget his lines in rehearsal. It is another thing altogether, becoming embarrassing often to the point of threatening, when it occurs in a performance. It is still more significant when the error results from the actor's own inadequate preparation. Rehearsals, after all, are intended to provide the preparation necessary to ensure that lines are not forgotten on opening night. They are the training ground in which competent practice is developed and tested. On stage, however, the rules change. One's reputation is at stake, as is the overall success of the production. One actor's lines are dependent upon the successful delivery of those that precede them. When the awkward pause created by a dropped line becomes palpable to the audience, the actor begins to sweat. It quickly becomes clear whose line was missed. As the pause lengthens, the embarrassment grows until the heat from the stage lights is overwhelming and all the watching eyes have burned holes through the actor's body. Although the moment is sure to pass eventually—the other actors will cover through ad-lib and improvisation—the moment has become etched in the memories of audience and cast alike. Of course, the moment is always more pronounced and long-lived for the actor than for the audience. While the audience is free to move with the cast to the next scene, for the actor, the incident replays like a scratched record. It is a small step for the embarrassment of the mistake to become the humiliation of personal failure.

Such humiliation formed the high point of this variation for many participants. Their reaction to the experience of not-knowing is different from merely feeling embarrassed. While embarrassment carries a connotation of something accidental and forgivable, humiliation indicates a personal failing, something of which one should be ashamed. There is something inside the terms that indicates duration as well. Embarrassment is accompanied by a red-faced chuckle and a mumbled apology. Very shortly, the incident which gave rise to it may become the punch line of a shared joke. Humiliation, on the other hand, is far less fleeting. Linked to personal failing, it is the companion of depression, of a lingering sense of shame, often the result of something that could have been prevented but was not. Forgetting one's lines is possibly cause for embarrassment; neglecting to prepare adequately and therefore compromising an entire production is humiliating.

For the stage actor, there is a clear distinction between embarrassment and humiliation. It is a given that, on occasion, lines will be dropped on the stage. It happens and, for the most part, it is not cause for humiliation. Youth workers, however, operate under the implicit professional assumption that not-knowing *must not* happen (or at least not to me). Even at our best, when we recognize that no one can possibly avoid all moments of stuckness, youth workers believe increased skill yields a decrease in these experiences. It becomes a direct relationship: The better the youth worker, the fewer these moments. The (albeit faulty) corollary follows shortly: experiences of not-knowing indicate less skillful practice and a less competent youth worker. Possibly due to the moral component of our work, we hold ourselves to a supercompetent standard that does not allow for lines to be missed. We assume that any time a failing occurs, it is the result of our ineptitude, of some failing on our part to do our jobs as well as others would do them. It is experienced as an indicator of incompetence, and it is grounds for humiliation.

When this occurred in a public setting, youth workers described crumbling under the weight of humiliation. When it took place in private, they talked about the paralyzing fear of what would happen when their peers and supervisors would discover their failing. Even describing their experiences many years after the fact, in the safety and anonymity of our interviews, youth workers felt shaken by the shame and humiliation of their experiences of not-knowing. Cleve's voice shook as she shared her narrative, connecting this experience with a social disaster whose magnitude can only be fully grasped in the context of the middle school social drama:

> It's stressing me out, thinking about it [nervous cough and laughter]. My throat's getting tighter... my chest is getting tight. It was the worst. It was just the worst public humiliation... worse than having my skirt rip on me in shop class in seventh grade.

Returning to the language of the stage, another worker, Stella, gives voice to a similar issue. She described the discomfort of what she perceived to be a spotlight on her at the height of not-knowing. She said, "It was like, essentially... all of a sudden she took that spotlight and put it on me.... I'm trying to figure out how to get the spotlight off me." For Stella, uncertainty in center stage became too uncomfortable to manage, but at the same time, she could do nothing about it. Like her peers described in previous themes, Stella's attention became concentrated on trying, in vain, to stop the experience. It gradually became myopic, allowing little or no awareness other than the heated shame of humiliation, a frantic urge to scramble off-stage, and an inability to find a means of making that escape.

A final feature of the participants' humiliation came from the fear that by not knowing what to do, they had caused harm to other people. This is the connection between the actor and the rest of the cast, the dropped line and the integrity of the entire production. As with the sensation of helplessness and futility expressed in the previous theme, youth workers described their humiliation as coming from their inability to respond to the needs of their clients. Stephanie and Eve talked about feeling ashamed of their inactivity at precisely the moment their clients needed them the most. For Stephanie, attacked and uncertain of how to soothe her aggressive client, this reflected her failure as a youth worker. She described leaving the facility after her shift, uncertain whether she would return and doubting whether she could show her face in the group home again. Eve's reaction was similar, governed by an overwhelming sense of personal failing: "There's that sense of shame, y'know? 'What's wrong with me?'" This speaks again to the myth of supercompetence, under which youth workers accept that they must always be able to help. It may be a defense against their anticipation of the futility (discussed in the previous chapter) of not always being able to help. In any case, their humiliation came from these youth workers' beliefs that they had failed and were, themselves, failures as youth workers. Having failed, in their minds, to respond to their clients' needs was worthy of shame. It was a humiliating defeat and, in their eyes, it was a defeat from which their clients suffered.

THEY'LL KNOW I'M A FRAUD

The humiliation of being unable to respond gives shape to the experience of exposure and vulnerability that makes up this theme's second variation. Youth workers described feeling completely vulnerable in the moment of not-knowing, partially because of the feeling of being under the spotlight or in center stage and partially due to the sense of having their defenses stripped away. The latter, discussed in the previous chapter, is a general feature of not-knowing; it intersects with several themes. The former speaks to the root of this variation: youth workers identified feeling on display, exposed in what they perceived to be their incompetence.

Vulnerability is implied in the very concept of exposure. After all, being exposed carries very specific connotations. Different from merely being out in the open, being exposed implies the presence of a viewer or potential viewer. To be exposed, something that might otherwise be hidden must be seen. Exposure indicates that what was once covered or protected has been laid bare. For instance, in carpentry or home improvement, one speaks of exposed beams in a ceiling. The beams are *exposed* precisely because, contrary to most beams that are hidden by a plaster ceiling, these have no such cover. Connecting to the theme of helplessness in the moment of not-knowing, this sense of exposure resonates with the erosion of a youth worker's defenses. As the beams are exposed when their plaster covering is removed, so is the youth worker exposed once his defenses have worn away. This was certainly true for Cleve: "Exposure . . . y'know, [it's] about me . . . not being able to defend myself. That's really frustrating. And that was kind of the underlying feeling in the moment." Her sense of exposure indicated not only that her not-knowing (which she experienced as failure) was on display, but that she had no defenses to manage it.

In general, when youth workers spoke of feeling exposed, they identified clear elements of themselves that had been made public. For the most part, participants talked about having their incompetence exposed through the moment of not-knowing. Like Chris in the vignette, they became certain that everyone witnessing their moment of uncertainty knew them to be incompetent and interpreted their inactivity as reflective of a personal and professional failing. This is the root of the humiliation described in the previous variation. Again and again, I heard participants measure themselves against a youth work ideal that smacked of the unrealistic supercompetence they believed to be personally unattainable but universally fulfilled by their peers. In other words, youth workers assumed that although they could never meet such a goal, their colleagues possessed the competence and skill repertoire to anticipate and respond effectively to any situation they might encounter. Even when they thought somewhat poorly of actual peers, they held themselves to this standard of comparison to an abstracted or idealized notion of their colleagues and their skill.

Perceiving themselves to be fundamentally inadequate to this task, youth worker participants expressed their most humiliating moments as those when their inadequacies were exposed to their peers. As with some of the previous themes, the anticipation of this moment was, for many, as bad as the moment itself. Throughout the experience of not-knowing, for instance, Vanessa remembered being consciously afraid of being "found out" by her supervisors, graduate instructors, peers, and even her clients. Seeing herself as a fraud masquerading as a competent youth worker, she (like many other participants) became burdened by the weight of her own perceived failing, rather than mustering the strength to debunk the myth of supercompetence.

None of the youth workers who experienced this exposure of incompetence questioned whether they were, in fact, incompetent. On the contrary, it was accepted as a given, in the moment, that not knowing what to do was not an indicator of an unmanageable situation but, rather, an illustration of their fundamental inadequacy. Like the image on an undeveloped photo negative, their failings existed, merely awaiting exposure. Cleve's experience of not-knowing reinforced the fear that she might be exposed: "[I go] around pretending that I know what I'm doing. And [if] people find out that I really don't... they would think I'm a big sham." The fear of being "found out," in Vanessa's words, became paralyzing, as youth workers began to question what would happen to them once their supervisors or peers knew them to be charlatans.

The dominant feature of this self-perception is not the vocational question of one's worth or ability to do youth work. On the contrary, it is the fundamental assumption that although the youth worker is in the right line of work, he will never be anything other than a fraud in the eyes of *real* youth workers. Incompetence is a foregone (and self-perpetuating) conclusion. This is not the fear of being incompetent. That fear is the source of larger questions of calling and vocation that are discussed in the next chapter. On the contrary, it is the fear of having one's existing incompetence discovered. Like the impending doom of watching one's defenses crumble, the anticipatory shame associated with being publicly shown to be a fraud is enough to paralyze the youth worker. The distinction drawn here illustrates the extent to which youth workers accept the myth of supercompetence as true and remain bound by its requisite comparisons, judging themselves and their practice against an idealized, impossible, and in the absence of authentic dialogue about the intersections of self and practice, fundamentally abstracted peer.

As Vanessa, Ophelia, Eve, and others described in their interviews and as Chris's story in this chapter's opening vignette makes clear, the uncertainty of what might ensue as the outcome of this exposure is as paralyzing as the experience itself. Throughout her narrative, Vanessa returned to this question, recalling her anxiety of being found out and the potential disciplinary action that might follow. Ophelia described never talking about her experience with her colleagues—part of a cultural norm in the agency that suggested that line staff would do well not to have their supervisors know about such moments of uncertainty. Resulting from a self-perception of incompetence and inadequacy in the face of a youth work ideal, fear of exposure—not introspective examination of the experience—is the hallmark of this variation.

Chapter 8

It's Just a Little Too Human: Questions of Vocation

SUMMARY. Among youth workers who experience moments of not-knowing what to do, many often describe their thoughts and reactions to the phenomenon in vocational and existential terms. They ask what right they have to work in the helping professions if they find themselves simply unable to be helpful. In many cases, the vocational crises following experiences of not-knowing contribute to burnout and youth workers' decisions to leave the field altogether. This chapter describes the fourth of five themes associated with youth workers' experiences of not knowing what to do: questions of vocation. In addition to presenting the dominant theme, this chapter discusses the three variations on it, as described by youth worker participants: (a) What am I supposed to do? (b) Who am I to deal with this? and (c) Maybe the problem is me.

VIGNETTE: THE WEIGHT OF THE WORLD

Looking across the table at Erin, there was a sense of uncertainty in the back of my mind about what in the world I was doing there. I had been working with her for the past several weeks, since her state social worker contacted me to say that if things didn't change, Erin was going to be expelled from school and moved from her foster home into a more restrictive group care setting. Her behavior in both places was out of control—loud and defiant, although not violent—and the pressure was on me to help her figure out how to do things differently. If I didn't get through to her, I was told, she would be moved. Who knew what would happen then.

The problem was that Erin wasn't exactly communicative. She said she wanted to keep meeting with me, but when we actually sat down together, nothing happened. She refused to talk. We would spend an hour just staring at one another, with me asking questions, trying every trick I knew to get her engaged. She would just stare, arms crossed, until it was time to go, and then ask if she could come back next week. At this particular coffee date, I remember thinking that the stakes were higher than they had been; if we weren't able to make significant progress in a very short period of time, Erin's life would soon change in ways she was not likely to enjoy.

Looking across at her, I knew she was aware of what was planned for her unless things changed. Her eyes were puffy and red, she looked like she hadn't been sleeping, but she still wouldn't talk. Knowing something about her history, I knew Erin must have been in incredible emotional pain. But I didn't know what to do to help her. I mean, I know that it's not my job to fix people's lives for them. I have to trust that the kids I work with have the power to run their own lives. At the same time, she obviously needed something, some reassurance from someone. She was used to being so tough in front of everyone, I thought, quite honestly, that if I could just reach across the table and hug her, cry with her, give her permission to be vulnerable, she just might make it.

I was torn. I knew what I *wanted* to do. I knew what would be helpful to do. But I didn't know what I *should* do. Professionally, I mean. Because I knew I was on the edge.... I was close to ignoring my professional roles or boundaries, to responding to what, in my gut, I thought she needed, even though it might not have been the right thing to do therapeutically. It felt horrible—like I was being pulled in several directions. I felt like I was being drawn and quartered—wanting to give her the personal, human connection I thought she needed but being pulled in the opposite direction by my feelings of obligation to maintain a professional image. That's where I felt the most stuck: What was I supposed to do? Staring at her, having her puffy eyes staring back, I wanted to just make all the difficulty go away for her. But I didn't know how.

And then, in the middle of it all, I heard the social worker's voice over and over in my head, reminding me that it was up to me to figure out how to help Erin. The pressure to live up to these expectations became overwhelming—everyone expected me to know how to fix her, and I didn't even know where to begin. I felt stupid and embarrassed; everyone else thought I knew what to do, so I was probably supposed to know what to do. But I didn't. It was intimidating. Intimidating and frustrating. How *could* I know what to do?! I was only one part of her world, and she hadn't even chosen (of her own accord) to share anything about herself with me! How much control could I really have over the outcome of our time together?! I was being turned into the uninformed expert! It was just too much all at once, the realization that I had been given so much power over this young woman's life. It felt uncomfortable. It just didn't fit. Everyone put the weight of the outcome on me, but I wasn't the one who had to live with the consequences. I had too much influence over her future! I just wanted out!

Sitting there, staring at Erin's blank face—not feeling like I knew what to do or when to do it or what tone to even say it in—felt like it was just way too powerful. Having that much power scared me. I was in a position that I didn't deserve to be in, but I couldn't figure out how to get out of it! I worried that I didn't know how to handle the situation and that my uncertainty would cause Erin to be hurt. My heart started racing really fast, like it was stuck somewhere in my throat, like it does when you have to stand up and speak in front of a crowd. My mind started working overtime, forecasting down the road: "Well, if I fail now (because that's what it would have been—my failure as a youth worker), then two weeks from now, it's going to be that much worse for her." And, worst of all, I'm going to become just another one in the long string of adults who have let her down. Everything started to look negative, bleak, and it was all because I couldn't live up to the expectations put on me. Because I couldn't do my job.

I remember that I started to squirm at some point—actually fidgeting in my chair. I felt totally overwhelmed, a feeling like, "I can't do this. I don't want to do this." The whole world zoomed in on our table, and it occurred to me that maybe I was never meant for youth work. Maybe I was having such a hard time because it was a mistake for me to be in the field at all. After all, this was hardly an emergency. It was actually a fairly routine situation but, for some reason, it had brought me to my knees. I wanted to surrender, to admit that I didn't know what I was doing, that I was a fraud, and that I had no place working with kids. All I could think about was running away. But what would that mean about me? What would that say about me as a person, not just as a youth worker? I would be a failure. I would have to admit defeat. I would have to admit that I had no right to do this work. Who would I be then? Staring at Erin, with these questions in my mind, I felt lost—just completely lost with no way of knowing how to get home.

IT'S JUST A LITTLE TOO HUMAN

Where other themes concerned youth workers' experiences of themselves in the moment of not-knowing and emphasized the embodied, in-the-now descriptions of not-knowing itself, this theme focuses on the meanings participants made of the experience during and after the fact. More reflective than descriptive, it revolves around the effects of not-knowing in and after the situation in which it occurred. The theme revolves around youth workers' perceptions—including their struggles, questions, and attitudes—toward their professional identities.

Despite how many times frustrated clients may accuse them of it, youth workers are seldom in the field just because "It's a job." On the contrary, they talk about being called to the profession, feeling compelled in some way to commit their lives to working with and on behalf of young people. The concept of vocation or calling, having come from and found its most fertile soil in religious discourse (and youth work in religious communities), has also made its way into the helping professions, and it is the draw for many people entering the field. It sustains many youth workers (and the youth with whom they work) through difficult personal and professional moments; it represents and reinforces the moral component of the profession. While it resonates with many youth workers, warming their hearts and providing direction for their vocational lives, the sense of moral commitment also holds the potential to introduce significant emotional pain, existential struggle, and vocational doubt.

This theme turns to some of these struggles. Three variations emerged to give shape to the theme. The first two focus on youth workers' questions about and conflicts with their professional roles in the context of not-knowing. The first variation, "What am I *supposed* to do," concerns youth workers' binary identity, the divide they perceive between their personal and professional selves. Although the field prides itself on encouraging the active integration of the personal with the professional, youth workers often find the two identities in conflict with one another. Nowhere is this conflict more evident than in moments of not-knowing.

The second variation concerns youth workers' experiences of power and the discomfort associated with its use. Often, participants described finding themselves in situations where they became aware that they wielded a significant amount of power or influence over certain features of their clients' lives, and they felt uncomfortable in these positions. This discomfort became more pronounced in moments of not-knowing, as youth workers struggled to reconcile an external demand for the effective use of their power with their own inability and uncertainty to direct it appropriately.

The final variation stands as a category of its own. Concerning the larger questions of calling and purpose that arose in youth workers' reflection on their experience of not-knowing, this variation contains many features of the themes presented in the previous three chapters. The vocational questions associated with calling or purpose, and the crises in vocation that emerge in and after the moment of not-knowing, cut across the other themes while also growing out of them. They are questions raised consistently by participants in reflecting on their experiences of not-knowing, and they speak to the very core of the youth work profession.

What Am I Supposed to Do?

Throughout the interview process, and in subsequent conversations with professionals in the field, I have been struck by how often I hear youth workers describe themselves in purely binary terms. Several participants in the original study, particularly when discussing the vocational questions surrounding their experiences of not-knowing, talked about feeling torn between two halves of themselves: their personal or human selves and their professional selves. The idea that the two were distinct identities was troubling but not surprising for me. That the personal and professional selves differ and should be kept separate has long been accepted in the helping professions. After all, the image of the classical psychoanalyst reflects the understanding that therapists' personal lives must be divorced from their professional practice, lest issues of transference and countertransference interfere with (rather than complement) treatment. In education and social work, youth work's parent disciplines, these lines are somewhat fuzzier but present nonetheless. Both fields encourage the maintenance of clear boundaries between the personal and professional (and therefore, between social worker and client, or teacher and student), but they allow more flexibility than classic psychiatry or psychology.

As an emerging profession, American youth work prides itself on the integration of these personal and professional selves. Youth workers are trained to see themselves as operating somewhere in the middle of the spectrum, neither bound by the austere starkness of the blank slate nor the blurred boundaries of the best friend. They function in the middle, balancing both worlds at once and attempting to fulfill the obligations demanded by each. Although this is particularly true in many types of residential care, it is not limited to these environments; religious youth work, street outreach, and chemical dependency treatment present further examples. Nevertheless, maintaining this binary, seeing themselves as constantly walking the line between their personal and professional selves, demands much conscious energy. Preserving authentic connection while also remaining professionally detached can be exhausting for youth workers.

Each identity, personal and professional, makes significant and discrete demands on the youth worker, and participants described the moment of not-knowing as characterized by a feeling of being caught between these demands. On one hand, previous themes have addressed youth workers' perceived needs to maintain a professional veneer in their work, both for their own benefit and on behalf of their clients. On the other, the profession's moral imperative—to walk carefully and sensitively with youth—often demands that youth workers deliberately bring their emotions and values to the forefront of their work. Presenting the emotional self in this context can be both powerful and threatening for youth workers. It can create a double-bind for youth workers in that their desire to connect with their clients in a meaningful and authentic way (potentially exposing the personal or emotional self) may run counter to their agencies' policies or guidelines governing self-disclosure, attachment, and the like. This became, for many, the height of stuckness, as they anticipated the conflict but saw no way of resolving it so that both interests were satisfied. They felt forced to choose.

Caught in this way, between her initial emotional connection and her professional expectations, Stella found herself uncertain of how to reconcile this double-bind. Sitting across from a client who begged her for the disclosure Stella wanted to offer (and knew would be helpful to the youth), she said, "There was one moment . . . where it was kind of like [a sense of] discovery and elation at just a human connection . . . and then the next moment was, 'Oh shit! I'm in a professional role here. What do I do'" Like Stella, youth workers often find themselves in situations where their professional or organizational obligations force them to suppress the initial emotional instincts and reactions of their personal selves.

The conflict between these identities became the dominant feature of not-knowing for many youth workers. In contrast to the issues of professionalism evident in the discussion of helplessness and the lack of control, which concerned how youth workers maintained their professional veneer in moments of not-knowing, this variation presented a different question. The vocational question participants faced in this regard was, initially, whether they should preserve that veneer, erring on the side of their professional obligations when doing so would require the stifling of their emotional and personal reactions. In most cases, youth workers knew what they, personally, wanted to do in response to the immediate situation, but their experience of not-knowing came in their uncertainty about what they, professionally, *ought* to do. Again, Stella's experience speaks loudly: "[I was] feeling that clash between the personal, human responsibility and your responsibility as an employee and as a [youth worker]." While she could name the conflict—what she called the "clash"—she struggled to resolve it. Expanding on Stella's experience, Lori described feeling torn between her personal need to grieve with her clients and her perceived professional obligation to remain stoic and strong, creating an environment where they could grieve in their own ways.

Lori's experience points to the first of several features of this uncertainty that warrant further discussion. First, her situation presupposed that a right answer existed and that this right answer was rooted in the professional (not personal) identity. Based on the presumption that as professionals, there is an imperative, something they *should* do, participants like Lori struggled between behaving competently as youth workers and responding compassionately as human beings. To do the latter signified, to them, a failure to do the former.

For Athena, hugging her client and assuring him that she absolutely did believe God loved him may have been the most compassionate response, but it could have represented a significant breach of her obligation as his youth worker. Athena's moment of not-knowing became crystallized around whether to allow her heart or her head to direct her response: "I didn't know what I was 'supposed' to say, from an agency perspective, but . . . from a human perspective, it's like, 'Of course, God loves you'" Torn between her personal connection with this young person and the professional context in which that connection occurred, Athena spoke as though conscious that the answer she wanted to give was not the answer she was expected to give.

Second, participants shared the sense that they were alone in their uncertainty; other youth workers would know precisely how to manage these competing interests. Echoing the dynamic of their peers' supercompetence in the face of their own ineptitude (addressed in greater detail in the previous theme), youth workers described the anxiety associated with their uncertainty. In this way, not-knowing was not merely a failure to meet the demands of their personal interests. More significantly, it created a conflict in terms of their sense of themselves as effective youth workers. Feeling forced to choose between attending to personal or professional interests, they found themselves required to affirm one and deny the other—a position that ran counter to the ideal conception of youth work as the effective integration of professionalism and human engagement.

The participants began to question the larger vocational issues involved: what would it mean for them as caring and compassionate people if they failed to respond personally to what they perceived to be the human needs their clients presented? At the same time, what would it mean for them as professionals if they were unable to bracket their personal reactions sufficiently to respond in a way that appeared professionally competent? Drizzt said, "If I were good at my job, I would have been able to solve this problem," indicating that the struggle to integrate these halves of himself is only a struggle because of his professional inadequacy.

It is significant in their descriptions of this experience that youth workers found no middle ground among these questions. They could see no way, in the moment, of integrating the two positions, responding professionally and still compassionately (or responding personally within a certain set of professional guidelines). On the contrary, they felt forced to choose one over the other and, in so doing, became paralyzed and unable to do either well. At any other moment, this integration might present no challenge, but in the experience of stuckness, no resolution was possible. Not-knowing how to resolve the tension between the two, youth workers were left adrift in the push-pull of this vocational question: What am I *supposed* to do?

Who Am I to Deal with This?

In addition to the vocational dilemma posed by conflicts between their personal and professional selves, a number of youth workers identified a profound discomfort with the power of their positions, which became most glaring during the moment of not-knowing. American youth workers, accustomed to seeing themselves as partners with youth, often do not give conscious attention to the positional power they actually hold vis-à-vis their clients. In fact, they often see themselves directly in opposition to the status quo, working with and on behalf of their clients against a set of oppressive social service powers that be. Aligning themselves with their clients in contrast to more established professions (social work is often key among these), youth workers unintentionally obscure the fact that they actually do carry a significant amount of authority by virtue of their positions.

In some cases, the recognition that they hold this power is a startling and promising realization for youth workers. After all, if used correctly, such power may open doors that would otherwise remain closed for their clients. If, however, the youth worker is uncertain how to exercise this power, it can quickly become overwhelming. Further, in a field whose rhetoric encourages youth workers to see young people as possessing power and authority over their own lives, to be put in a position of holding power or significant decision-making authority over a client (particularly without the client's participation or active buy-in), is vocationally troubling. As illustrated in the vignette and throughout many participants' interviews, this was not merely a discomfiting situation. On the contrary, it introduced significant vocational questions related to a profound ethical quandary concerning the just and unjust uses of authority.

It is one thing to possess and use power we have come to hold through legitimate means (or through means we determine to have been legitimate). In these cases, the exercise of authority and power are not only acceptable, they can be ethically obligatory. Likewise, even in a field where power is often treated as a dirty word, youth workers mention feeling comfortable using their authority when they are confident in how it is best used: advocating for a young person before a sentencing judge, using credentials and position to vouch for a young person's character or employability, or using professional relationships and channels to ease a youth's social service transitions are clear examples of this just use of authority. If either of these conditions—the just acquisition and intentional direction—is absent, however, the experience of finding oneself in a position of authority can become overwhelming.

In the moment of not-knowing, youth workers described becoming aware of their power in the absence of both criteria. They neither felt themselves to have earned the power they held nor knew how they were to use it effectively or responsibly. Expected to make residential placement recommendations for a client who was only marginally invested in her or their work together, Vanessa questioned both her right to possess the power she held and how she ought to use it in service of her client. She said, "[I was] feeling like I had no way to reach out to this child, feeling like [I had] a lot of power, and I really don't know what I'm doing. That scares me." Lacking a clear sense of what she had done to earn her privileged position vis-à-vis her client, she also had no idea how to leverage that position in her client's best interests. At the same time, however, she and the other youth workers who shared this experience were aware of being expected (by clients, parents, or other professionals) to know what to do and to act effectively on that knowledge: "Other people are looking at me to be the expert who has the answers [and I have nothing]." The pressure to act mounted as, like Vanessa, participants became increasingly aware of the expectation that they would rise to the challenge. This pressure was heightened by two distinct questions, echoing the criteria mentioned earlier, that seemed to run on a loop through youth workers' minds.

Vanessa and Athena both spoke with a tone of desperation and fear of their discomfort holding such power. They, like others, wondered: What does it mean if I mess up with this much power? The pressure to act and fear of action was exaggerated, for many youth workers, by their awareness of the potential outcome of their decisions for the youth involved. As Vanessa's narrative illustrated, it was difficult for youth workers to reconcile themselves to the authority they had been given to make decisions with far-reaching implications for their clients. This was bad enough. Even worse was the realization that, despite the long-term consequences of their decisions, they had no idea how to appropriately manage the situations over which they had been given such authority. It is at this point that the discomfort with their positional power became a vocational dilemma. Youth workers began to question not only what it meant for themselves that they had no idea how to respond but, also, what it would mean, in the long run, for their clients. Thinking about the outcome of her recommendation on her client and with watering eyes, Vanessa asked, "Can my conscience live with . . . that . . . for the rest of his life?" For months after her experience of not-knowing, Sweet Pea remembered feeling a similar worry, dreading the news that her indecision had permanently hurt the youth with whom she worked.

The concern for the clients is obvious; caring for the other is one of the hallmarks of the profession and a key reason why people enter the field in the first place. As such, it is hardly surprising that youth workers would worry about the effects of their not-knowing on the youth with whom they work. But the vocational question was as significant: Who am *I* to deal with this? Why has this fallen in *my* lap? Voicing these questions, Ophelia said, "I didn't want to [manage this situation]. It felt tainted, a little bit. I just felt like, 'Why do *I* have to do this? Why do *I* have to witness this?!'" Believing themselves, on some level, to be frauds (as described in the last chapter), youth workers struggled to make sense of what made them worthy of such power. Possessing power they did not believe themselves to have earned and being looked to for answers, they doubted their ability to give put youth workers in an uncomfortable vocational dilemma at a time when they were least prepared to answer or resolve it, paralyzed and myopic as they had become in the moment of not-knowing.

Maybe the Problem Is Me

While the first two variations concerning youth workers' confusion about their roles and discomfort with the power they carry relate to questions of *how* to do their work, the final variation relates to *whether* they should be doing this work in the first place. It is the heart-wrenching, soul-searching question of vocation in its purest form. Revolving around questions of calling, this feature is highly interpretive; it represents the meaning youth workers made of their stuckness, despair, helplessness, and hopelessness upon reflecting on the moment of not-knowing. Looking back over their experiences, youth workers often came to the conclusion—reminiscent of the myth of supercompetence—that they encountered these moments because of a fundamental flaw on their part. For some, the flaw represented professional incompetence, while for others it reflected their misinterpretation of their calling (or their purpose for being on the planet). Regardless of its origin, youth workers extrapolated from their experience the lesson that they had no place in the field. Drizzt said

> God! I thought I was a pretty good [youth worker], but I couldn't help these guys out. How many more of these am I gonna have? Am I gonna be cut out for this at all? For this line of work? Will I be able to do this? Can [I] keep doing this . . . if it keeps happening, this kind of situation comes up?

This is the issue of vocational crisis at its most extreme and, as Drizzt's question suggests, it may be the point of most significant burnout for youth workers.

Nearly all the participants described at least a brief moment, usually immediately after the experience of not-knowing, where they doubted their ability—in some cases, their right—to do youth work at all. Across the board, they attributed this doubt to their inability to act, again reflecting the myth of supercompetence described in the last chapter. They did not question that expectation, possibly because they assumed themselves to be the only youth workers struggling to attain it. On the contrary, they identified that the problem rested in their own laps and with their lack of skill. For them, the inability to respond reflected their inadequacy for the profession and, in some cases, the danger their incompetence presented for their clients.

For some, like Vanessa, this related to the human component of youth work. Echoing the binary split between personal and professional selves, Vanessa described feeling downtrodden by the experience of not-knowing, because even as she erred on the side of professional competence, she found the emotional toll of the experience to be too overwhelming. Knowing not only that she carried the weight of her own decisions on her shoulders, but also the results of those decisions for her client, Vanessa described the field as "too human" for her. She said, "[If I can't do this], am I really pursuing the career and the field that I should be pursuing? Because it doesn't feel like I should be in this place at this point. It's a little too human." Hers was a question of calling, of whether or not she should be in the field. It is as though her experience of not-knowing served as a mirror, reflecting how her professional life ought to look. Gazing from that mirror to her actual experience, Vanessa found her reality lacking in comparison to her ideal. As a result, she questioned herself—not the viability of the ideal.

Stephanie shared a similar set of vocational questions as she left the group home on the day of her experience of not-knowing. She had spent her workday attacked, bleeding, unassisted by her peers, and wondering how to make sense of the entire situation. Upon leaving the facility, she recognized that it was possible she was being tested—by the clients, by the other staff, and possibly by the world. As she walked out the door, a coworker jokingly asked whether she would be back the next day. Desperately wanting to pass the test, which would indicate her worth as a youth worker, Stephanie said yes. But, she said, "I cried in the car on the way home, just like 'You gotta be kidding!' Like all that stuff… getting more and more built up inside… and I'm finally like… 'I don't think I did very well. I don't know if I can do this.'" For her, like others, the experience became personalized; any difficulty resulted from her failing and must reflect on her ability to do her work.

Perhaps because of the moral component of their professional work, which is, after all, to help young people develop, youth workers often feel compelled to find a place in the field. Whether this is understood through the "world speaking," as one youth worker put it, or through the Christian notion of a call, or something else altogether, it brings a sense of dedication and purpose to the work. It is a devastating thing, then, for youth workers to see their inability to be helpful as an indication that they are unworthy of the call they thought they heard. For many, this leads to premature departure from the field. Stella and Eve, for example, left their positions shortly after their experiences of not-knowing. Neither knows whether or not she will return to the field. Vanessa learned from her experience that perhaps she was not "cut out" for youth work. Although still in the field, she occasionally wonders, "Maybe it was better to be an administrative assistant, because it's a lot less risky than this work . . . there are probably other people who could be doing this better than I am, and maybe I should get out while I can."

The weight of not-knowing is heavy and its meanings can be burdensome for youth workers. While for some these center around the discomfort associated with reconciling their personal and professional selves in their work, for others they have to do with the pressure brought by positional authority of which they do not feel deserving. They are desperate questions of vocation, as Ophelia's cry illustrates:

> It was just so scary and sad . . . like, Oh my god, here's a situation I can't handle. And what does that . . . what does that mean? You know? What does that . . . what does that mean about the world? What does that mean about me doing this work? I started to question myself and my abilities. You know? What are we doing this work for? Why am I doing this? Why this? Why not some other job?

Across the board, youth workers voiced these questions of vocation. They relate to youth workers' uncertainty about their field and the fundamental sense of themselves as worthy or unworthy of the profession's moral obligations, and although they cut to the youth worker's core, they are seldom answered.

Chapter 9

Not-Knowing Gives Way to Knowing

SUMMARY. One of the few truly reassuring features of not-knowing among youth workers is the realization that not-knowing cannot last forever. Eventually, some feature of the situation shifts, and youth workers move back into the capacity for action. This chapter describes the last of five themes associated with youth workers' experiences of not knowing what to do: Not-knowing gives way to knowing. In addition to presenting the dominant theme, this chapter discusses the three variations on it, as described by youth worker participants: (a) The rousing power of someone else, (b) I have to respond, because no one else will, and (c) The power of winging it.

VIGNETTE: IT JUMPSTARTED MY BRAIN

It had been such a successful outing that nobody was quite ready to go back home. I had taken seven teenagers, all on probation or parole, for an 8-mile hike in the hills, and we were headed back to their group home when someone suggested that, since they had been so good and since it was so hot, we should make a stop at the river so they could swim for a few minutes. It had sounded like a good idea at the time, so we wound up at Johnson's Eddy for a dip.

The swimming hole was pretty crowded, but we found a spot a bit away from other people and went over some ground rules. Right away, the kids started begging for permission to jump off the rocks on the other side of the river—rocks that were maybe 8 or 10 feet above the water. Other people were doing it, they said, so it must be safe. They argued that the water was obviously deep enough, and they promised me they could all swim. They had been really good all day, they reminded me. Didn't that mean they deserved a reward?

They were pleading with me, making me feel completely conflicted. I was really torn. On the one hand, the kids had a good point—other people *were* jumping off the rocks (I had, too, when I was a kid, and more than a little bit, I wanted to get in the water today just about as badly as they did), and they *had* had a great day. Why not? On the other hand, I was conscious of my own responsibility to keep them safe. I wasn't their parent and didn't feel comfortable giving them permission to do something so potentially dangerous. It was like the little cartoon angel on one shoulder and devil on the other. They both had good points. I didn't know which one to listen to. I was stuck between what I wanted and what I thought I was supposed to do.

I remember I just stood there, staring at them, wishing I had another adult there to help me make the decision. But I didn't. It was just me, and I didn't know what to do. I waffled. Then I started forecasting, conjuring up all the "what ifs" I could imagine for both responses. I could just see myself, 2 years down the road, finding out that one of the kids wound up with some horrible injury because I had let them jump. I was totally tormented by the thought of it. But at the same time, I felt deeply guilty about possibly telling them no.

I don't know how long I stood there, wavering back and forth, completely unsure of how I should respond. I just stared at them, my mind working overtime, trying to decide between the safe and prudent angel and the fun-loving devil. They all stared back at me, which was unnerving, pressuring. I had no response for them. It was an eternity of staring.

Then, out of nowhere, some guy I had never seen before walked up to our group, which must have looked pretty strange with everyone standing in a circle staring at one another. "Everything okay? Y'all need anything?" he asked. It was an innocent enough question, but it totally transformed the scene. That guy jumpstarted my brain.

It was like waking up! I think I just was so stuck in my own head that I needed something, anything, to shake me out of it. All of a sudden, I could see again. Things seemed clear, like when you leave the chiropractor's office and the whole world seems different—everything is sharper, clearer. It's like everything has been readjusted in the space of a moment. I don't think I even responded to the guy. It wasn't about him or what he said. It was just that I had stepped outside of the situation, outside of my head, and I could finally look at what was happening. It was enough to get me going again, to get me out of my head and back into the moment.

I realized that we couldn't stand there forever; somebody had to make a decision. That somebody was me! I could have stayed stuck like that for a long time if I hadn't come up with the discovery that I was the one in charge. Nobody else was coming to tell me what to do. Not that I knew what to do all of a sudden; I didn't. But I knew I had to do something. I had to make the call, one way or the other. That was weird. It was almost refreshing to realize that I *could* make the decision, that I had whatever I needed to make this call and I could deal with whatever came next. There was a little bit of relief, realizing that there was no choice, that I had to do something, and I had to trust that it was going to work out. I didn't really have a choice.

Like I said, I still didn't know what to do. I was still winging it, just kind of going off what I thought, in my gut, was probably the right thing to do. I let the kids jump. I felt really scared, almost panicky, when I told them they could go, but I also told them I wasn't totally sure this was the best decision. I was totally winging it, flying by the seat of my pants. If somebody had asked me to explain myself, I don't think I could have done it. That felt really risky, really dangerous. But at the same time, it felt kind of good not knowing what was coming next—it made me feel like the kids and I were on the same level in some way. Like neither of us knew what was happening, but we could figure it out together. I was still scared, but it didn't feel paralyzing. It felt open. Just really open.

NOT-KNOWING DOES NOT LAST FOREVER

Shortly after finishing the interviews for the original not-knowing study, I gave a presentation of the experience of not-knowing to a social work conference. As we discussed the themes of not-knowing midway through the workshop, someone (a current social work graduate student at a local university) raised her hand and said, "Man! This is depressing! You're making me wonder whether I should finish my degree!" Everyone in the room chuckled, including me, sharing a moment of collective agreement and understanding. Hers was an undeniable observation: the experience of not-knowing is a depressing one. But, as I assured this student, there is good news. Not-knowing ends.

Across the board, youth workers stressed that at some point in the experience, the pressure and paralysis of not-knowing gave way to something else. For all the participants, some moment occurred where they found themselves thrown back into their heads, so to speak, into the rational parts of themselves that allowed them to see that the experience could not last forever and that opportunities for action existed on the other side of it. This does not necessarily mean that youth workers immediately achieved the supercompetence they often held themselves responsible for possessing. They did not go immediately from the stuckness of not-knowing into action and effective crisis resolution. Instead, they returned to the point where not-knowing was no longer paralyzing. Not-knowing became one feature among many in the situations they faced; it was no longer the defining characteristic. Eventually, the moment of not-knowing itself passed, and youth workers talked about having returned to their "normal" professional lives.

For some, the first crack in the overwhelming stuckness of not-knowing came in the form of intervention by another person, often outside the event itself. In most cases, these people were completely uninvolved in the critical incident. In some cases (like the vignette), they were total strangers. This is not to say that these other people solved the problem or even, in most cases, provided useful insight into how it could be addressed. On the contrary, participants mentioned that merely having someone else present provided a sufficient interruption to their paralysis. For some, the interruption was merely another person walking into the room, completely unaware of the events unfolding there. For others, as in the vignette, it was someone asking something as simple as, "Are you okay?" Just as the circumstances giving rise to the moment of not-knowing were varied and often inconsequential to the actual experience, the details associated with being pulled out of the moment were, for the most part, insignificant. These people served a crucial function for the stuck youth workers: They expanded the workers' myopic perception, bringing the outside world back into what had been, until then, an entirely internal experience.

Others described coming out of the paralysis of not-knowing simply because they realized they had no other choice. Whether due to the passing of time, because of the realization that no one else could resolve the situation for them, or in light of their perceived professional duty to respond, these youth workers emerged from the cloud of not-knowing because no other options existed. Even when they did not know how, they had to respond in some way, lest their experience continue indefinitely. Although this realization often came more slowly than the immediate interaction or interruption of an outside voice, it nonetheless provided youth workers with a much-needed nudge back into action (or into the possibility of action).

A final group of participants talked very little about *how* they arrived at the realization that not-knowing would give way to something else. Instead, they described the meaning of that transition, from not-knowing to knowing, which they often came to understand only after the experience had passed. For youth workers in this group, not-knowing itself served as an invitation to openness. Not knowing what to do, in hindsight, freed these participants to consider doing things they would otherwise not have done. Further, it served as a leveling force between them and their clients, allowing them to experience something that was an everyday occurrence for the youth they served. In this way, the transition from not-knowing to knowing offered one group of participants a way of better understanding their professional practice—both as possibility and as connection.

Annie! Annie! Are You Okay? The Rousing Power of Someone Else

It is well known among crisis interventionists that at the moment of most urgent need, people are often too paralyzed to act. In many cases, some sort of distraction or intervention is required in order to shock people out of their indecision and create room for action. Following this logic, CPR workshops train interventionists to shout at the unconscious or choking victim and bark sharp and direct commands to onlookers. It is a common sight in social service agencies when the Red Cross or Health Department arrives for semiannual

CPR trainings: people shout at the plastic dummy on the floor, "Annie! Annie! Are you okay?!" And then to one another as onlookers: "You! Go call 911!" The power of an outside voice or the clear intervention of another person into moments of paralysis helps to shift people out of their heads and back into their bodies.

Several youth workers did not mention how they became aware of no longer being stuck in the moment of not-knowing, but for those who did, the realization often came with the introduction of someone else into the situation. In some cases, that someone else was a peer or colleague. In others, it was a stranger. In still others, it was a parent or the young people themselves. Regardless of who functioned as the someone else, that person represented an interruption in the paralysis of not-knowing (discussed in the first theme). In all cases, participants described their awareness of this other person's presence as freeing in some way.

For Ophelia, who experienced the stuckness of not-knowing in a very physical way, being attacked by a client while in a closed office with two other adults, the introduction of someone else into the situation "shook [her] out of a trance." It was her narrative that introduced the imagery of being like a deer in the headlights and, in discussing how she became aware of no longer not-knowing, she returned to that image. Finding herself paralyzed when her client began to attack first his mother and then her, all during a consultation involving the three of them and another professional, Ophelia described her mind as a complete blank. She felt entranced, able to see the immediate physical danger but betrayed by her body from doing anything about it. Like a deer in the headlights, she waited for the oncoming impact of the automobile. Time slowed and she became unable to focus on anything but the crisis.

She described that, at some point (possibly only seconds after the attack began, although she experienced it to have taken much longer), the other professional in the room looked at her and said, plainly, "Call 911." During our interview, Ophelia laughed at the simplicity of the instruction, but its effect on her was profound. Although the thought of calling 911 to interrupt an assault was not profound in itself, in the height of not-knowing, Ophelia could muster neither the thought nor physical energy required to complete the action. It took the intervention of another person, her colleague, to push her out of the paralysis into a position of action. She said, "When one person [has] the clarity to do whatever it is that they need to do, it's like suddenly you're . . . you've been awoken. I mean, that's what happened to me. I woke up out of the trance." The sense of having woken up is significant. Awakening, after all, creates nothing *new*. It merely dispels the dream and returns the sleeper to the place in which she fell asleep. Ophelia experienced nothing new, other than the return to what skills and awareness she had possessed prior to the incident's onset. She woke up—possibly still disoriented—but awake.

Lily described a similar sensation. Trying to work with a client whose housing was depending upon her assistance but who would not engage with her, Lily identified the crushing pressure associated with the stuckness of not-knowing. She, like Ophelia, not only felt unable to think of a response, she also could not will her body to move. This paralysis lifted when a coworker entered the room. Unlike Ophelia's situation, however, this coworker did not even speak; her presence in the room was sufficient to shake Lily out of the stuckness of not-knowing. Lily spoke of staring blankly at her client, waiting for something to happen that simply was not happening. The moment her environment shifted, however, by her colleague walking through the room, Lily regained her ability to act. It is as if, wrapped up in the myopic tunnel vision of the experience, participants found themselves unable to act. The moment that view became disrupted, however, as by the presence of another person, the paralysis of not-knowing lifted.

For Sweet Pea, the rousing power of someone else came from a complete stranger. Her experience served as the foundation for this chapter's vignette; her moment of not-knowing occurred in the context of deciding whether or not to allow her clients to jump off the rocks into a river swimming hole. Like Ophelia and Lily, she also described the physical stuckness of not-knowing, but hers resulted largely from out-of-body anchorlessness. Sweet Pea could not respond because she found herself without an anchor, without a foundation from which to act. Standing for some time paralyzed in not-knowing, she finally "snapped to" when a stranger down the riverbank announced that he was a lifeguard (and that, therefore, it would be safe for her to allow the youth to jump off the rocks). Describing this moment, Sweet Pea said she found an anchor in the stranger, even while consciously aware that he could have been lying (which would have invalidated her entire decision). His intervention, though actually insignificant and possibly dishonest, provided her with the foundation she needed in order to act.

Clearly, the power of these interventions came not in the advice they offered. After all, one said nothing at all, and another offered reassurance that may well have been a complete deception. Nor did it come in the degree to which they may have represented potential solutions to the immediate situation. Rather, these people's interruptions gave participants permission to act in spite of not-knowing. Breaking the sense of stuckness accompanying the experience, they allowed the youth workers to see that the moment of not-knowing was not eternal. This is not to say that the moment ended altogether and youth workers knew precisely what to do in response to the situation. Rather, they were merely no longer physically stuck in their bodies. Ophelia's description, that she had woken up, is telling. While stuck, she was unable to move or otherwise respond to her surroundings. Immediately upon waking, Ophelia and the other youth workers in the study found themselves again able to move but still disoriented. Coming out of the trance, or waking up, was the beginning of a process whose culmination is the full return of their faculties and ability to act. According to the participants, the first of these faculties to return was the realization that the moment could not last forever, and that they *could* act.

I Have to Respond Because There's No One Else

Many youth workers talked about the experience of not-knowing feeling eternal. In the moment, paralyzed by uncertainty, they described being unable to see an outcome—any outcome—to the situation. Although upon reflection, they realized that the moment actually took very little time, their lived experience of it was drawn out and seemingly endless. Vanessa described the stretching-out of time with a common metaphor: "It was kind of like watching a pot of water and waiting for it to boil . . . like every minute was at least five minutes." Others in the field have said that this perception resonated with their experiences of not-knowing as well; I heard from several social work conference participants that in the moment of not-knowing, they had no sense of when or how the experience would end. It was, in Lily's words, "an eternal moment."

Somewhere along the way, though, participants and others said that they became aware that despite how long it *seemed* to last, the moment simply could not continue forever. At some point, it must give way to action. At some point, the youth worker must be shaken out of the paralysis of not-knowing. While the presence of another person served this purpose for many participants, others said the permission to act came from a realization of their own isolation. In the context of the previous chapters, it seems almost contradictory that the realization of isolation could function not only as a paralyzing force but also as a liberating one. Nonetheless, many youth workers said they realized that not-knowing would end only when they became aware that they could not simply wait for someone else to act on their behalf. It was, for some, as though they had to sit in their own paralyzed isolation long enough to realize that waiting, by itself, would not bring resolution to the crisis.

With no one else to help them resolve the crisis or provide them with a sense of how to manage their situations, these youth workers recognized that although they did not know what, they had to do *something*. A conference participant put it similarly, saying, "You realize that you must respond." It struck me immediately that this statement carried two different connotations depending upon which words receive emphasis, and that both connotations shed light on the realization. Phrased as "You realize that *you* must respond," the statement refers to the youth worker's isolation in the timeless moment. Although the moment seemed like it could last forever, at some point the participants realized that they—and only they—had the power to bring it to an end. No one else would be coming to resolve the situation for them. Stella described the moment when she first realized that it was incumbent upon her to respond:

> There's this moment when everything goes blank and you realize you're the one in charge. You step outside of the situation and you look at yourself and you realize, "Uh-oh. I'm the one that's got to come up with the next step."

In general, participants did not describe this as a particularly comforting realization. Instead, it was initially somewhat worrisome. After all, Stella described it as an "uh-oh" moment. Although it carried the seeds of potential action, it was at once an affirmation of their isolation and a reminder of their responsibility to act effectively to resolve the situation (brought by the demands of their professional roles). For many, this realization brought back the pressures discussed earlier—both the vocational questions associated with the youth worker's power and the potentially crushing pressures imposed by the expectations of supercompetence. Still, despite being uncomfortable at first, for Stella and others, it was the first step toward moving through the moment of not-knowing.

The imposition of responsibility is best understood by repeating the conference participant's phrase with different emphasis. "You realize that you *must* respond" stresses that the youth worker has an obligation to respond. Again, this is the issue of the profession's moral imperative. There is a responsibility to resolve the immediate situation, and although this responsibility added to the pressure of the moment for many participants—as demonstrated in previous chapters—it served as an opportunity for others. Stella, for instance, saw in this realization an affirmation of her own competence. Its initial discomfort gradually gave way to a timid confidence. The moment reinforced for her that although she struggled with uncertainty, *she* was the adult present. *She* was the guide, the teacher, the youth worker. It was incumbent upon her to act, and she possessed, somewhere, the capacity to act. As if answering Ophelia's earlier description of herself as reduced to a powerless, childlike state in the moment of not-knowing, Stella's experience reverses this position, affirming her competence. Recognizing that she was a youth worker and carrying a professional moral obligation to serve her client, Stella was gradually pushed out of not-knowing and into something else. Still not quite *knowing*, Stella and others spoke of being moved into a place of being able to try, which—in the moment—was enough.

Athena described a similar experience, realizing that although she did not know what to do, she (and no one else) had an obligation to respond. For her, as well as for Stella, the realization brought a sense of relief and even of openness. Again, this is not to say that both immediately knew what they should do. Neither knew the appropriate course of action. Instead, the realization that they had to respond, both because there was no one else and due to their professional obligation, freed them from the paralysis they had previously experienced. It allowed them to start envisioning how to respond, returning them to the practical, reflective frame of mind that ultimately moved them through not-knowing.

The Power of Winging it

The final variation on this theme speaks to the openness of possibility that grew, for many youth workers, out of not-knowing.

Whether it came from the intervention of another person or through the realization that they had no choice *but* to respond, youth workers talked about a sense of openness that came with the end of not-knowing. As soon as they began to feel free from the pressure or stuckness of the moment, participants talked about the realization that not-knowing could be freeing. This point has been underscored by countless youth workers in presentations and classroom conversations. It is one of the points on which American youth work stakes its claim in the helping professions. We are free to be with youth, to encounter them on their own terms with few, if any, strings attached. For many, the movement out of stuckness reinforced this credo and brought it home in a new way.

Athena, for instance, described the transition from not-knowing to knowing as giving her permission to "wing it," suggesting that by embracing her own uncertainty, she created space to "fly by the seat of her pants" with her clients. Opening herself to the power of intuition that arose in the absence of rational strategy, she could envision possible courses of action that she might not have considered if she had not gone through the paralyzing experience of not-knowing. More specifically, she talked about the certainty of knowing what to do as a potentially limiting force, as confining as the stuckness encountered at the height of not-knowing. By contrast, the transitional point, where not-knowing began to give way to knowing, opened an opportunity for creativity and innovation. Further, Athena and Martin both talked about not-knowing as an experience that debunked their myths of supercompetence, demonstrating to them that they *could not* be expected (or expect themselves) to know immediately how to respond to every situation they might encounter. Unburdened by the weight of this expectation, Athena said the experience "felt kind of open. It actually felt open."

Building on that sense of openness, Stella suggested that although she "wasn't sure what direction to take or to steer the youth," she "felt like [she] had the capacity of figuring this out on [her] own." Athena shared a similar sense of her own capacity: "[I'm] going to go somewhere here [with my client], and I don't know where it is. I don't know where I'm going to go, but we'll get there." For the first time in their narratives, youth workers began to describe the emerging sense of possibility on the other side of not-knowing. What Athena called "winging it" introduced for the youth workers a sense of their own capacity in the midst of, not outside of, their uncertainty.

Although it had not been pleasant in the moment, on reflection, not-knowing served as an opportunity for exploration that was new to many participants.

Recognizing that they did not know what to do not only opened the door for them to consider doing things they otherwise might not have, it also allowed them to more fully join with their clients. As Athena mentioned, young people who come into services most often spend much of their time in their own experience of not-knowing. They often do not know how to navigate the complexities of the social service system nor, in many cases, do they know what to expect from the adults who come in and out of their lives. Theirs is an experience of chronic uncertainty. Athena talked about her own moment of not-knowing as a leveling phenomenon, one that exposed her, even if only for a brief time, to what her clients experienced on a regular basis.

As suggested earlier, reflecting on that experience allowed Athena to arrive at the integrated position youth work, as a field, aspires to: the blended personal and professional identity. Understanding first-hand how it felt to be uncertain in a situation where she believed she *ought* to have known what to do helped her to see herself in the experiences of her clients. She said the experience helped her to better join with them: "Me being in a position of 'I don't know what I'm going to do' just kind of balances us. And then we walk together." Although not all the participants came to this point of integrated reflection on the experience, Athena's realization nonetheless speaks to some of the power of "winging it," of knowing that she did not know and still mustering the strength to continue.

Chapter 10

So What? Now What? Implications for Youth Work Practice

SUMMARY. Youth work is a profession in development, engaged in the creation and practical application of its own theoretical base. This chapter connects the theoretical discussion and description of not-knowing to recommendations for practical action. Four lessons learned from the research are presented: (a) not-knowing is normal; (b) not-knowing cannot be prevented and need not be avoided; (c) the problems associated with not-knowing are more directly caused by youth workers' adherence to the myth of supercompetence; and (d) phenomenology offers a useful model for expanding youth work practice. From these lessons, recommendations are provided for front-line youth workers, supervisors, and the development of the profession as a whole.

I approached this study with the goal of better understanding a feature of my field that nearly all youth workers experience at some point in their careers but very few openly discuss. I wondered how my peers experienced moments of not-knowing and what meanings they made of these moments after they passed. I wondered what this exploration would teach me about my field, its role in the helping professions, and its ongoing struggles or challenges. During the study and through subsequent discussions and workshops with youth workers and other helping professionals about its findings, I have heard countless narratives of not-knowing and what it has meant for workers in the field.

As I analyzed and reflected on these stories and the contexts in which they emerged, I was struck by the richness and depth of understanding I found in their words. The participants' narratives provided glimpses into the moment of not-knowing as it was lived, allowing the reader to appreciate the questions, anxiety, excitement, and frustration of the experience. I have shared these descriptions with other youth workers who did not participate in the study and have consistently heard that these stories are much like their own. This is the hallmark of good phenomenology: the narratives and their interpretations help illuminate an experience that is shared but not often reflected upon.

Still, amid these colleagues' "aha!" moments, many questions arose. Several were immediately concerned with the practical and technical elements of this experience. Some workshop participants have commented that my presentations on not-knowing focused too much on the experience and asked what to *do* about the moment or how it can be prevented. Supervisors, in particular, have wanted me to identify some method or teach some tangible skill that will help them to ensure that their staff never encounter these experiences again.

Other questions concerned what I have come to call the myth of supercompetence and its meaning for youth work as an emerging profession. What does it mean for so many youth workers to operate under an expectation of perfection that allows little room for uncertainty or not-knowing? Can such a profession sustain itself? Can youth workers within that profession remain long in their careers? What does it mean for them either way? Others concerned a series of related questions about vocation and calling, which crystallized in one major concern: What does it mean about youth workers, personally and professionally, if they find themselves unable to live up to the expectations of their perception of the field's moral obligation?

Still other questions emerged about the utility of the methodology and the study itself. The interview in which they told their stories of not-knowing represented the first time many workers had shared these experiences in a way that felt supportive. Many reported that although they had played the events over and over in their minds and occasionally told their stories among friends in the spirit of comic relief, they had never honestly explored how they experienced these moments, what they meant at the time, and how they had shaped the workers' self-perceptions. These workers began to ask what role phenomenology could play in their work with young people, encouraging and providing a framework for deep exploration of experiences that might otherwise be ignored.

SO WHAT? LESSONS LEARNED

Several key lessons have emerged from reflection on these questions and the narratives that make up this study, each of which is relevant for practitioners, supervisors, and the emerging profession of youth work itself:

- Not-knowing is a normal and expected feature of work in the helping professions, and just because other youth workers may not talk about it does not make it any less real or legitimate.
- Not-knowing cannot be prevented and need not be avoided.
- Not-knowing is not the problem. Instead, the myth of supercompetence and its unrealistic expectations on youth workers makes these experiences problematic for the people living through them.
- Phenomenology as an interview method and theoretical orientation has much to offer youth work practice and supervision in the field.

Before addressing the practical applications of this study, each of these lessons warrants further explication.

NOT-KNOWING IS NORMAL

Perhaps the single most important and powerful lesson from this study is that not-knowing is a normal feature of work in the helping professions. It sounds deceptively simple and straightforward, and to many it seems as though this awareness ought to be self-evident. However, the interviews in this study and my conversations with youth workers in workshops and presentations argue to the contrary.

Workers routinely shared that they had no idea other people in their organizations or on their teams had experienced similar moments, largely because no one ever talked about them. Believing themselves to be the only staff to encounter moments of stuckness, these workers remained silent and continued to question and punish themselves for their perceived incompetence. For many, this silence grew into shame, and shame grew into a belief that they have no right to be in the field.

Many workers who experienced this profound sense of alienation, loneliness, and shame from not-knowing have commented that hearing from peers (whom they, across the board, believed to be competent) also struggled normalized the experience of not-knowing and affirmed the workers' own sense of skill and competence. Understanding that their peers also occasionally get stuck reinforces that not-knowing is simply another feature of youth work practice, as is a positive interaction or successful intervention with a young person. It is a liberating awareness.

Additionally, this study has taught that the events giving rise to moments of not-knowing vary from worker to worker and situation to situation. They are not always critical events, and the same circumstances that "stick" a youth worker in one moment may not in the next. Even so, many features of how the experience is lived are commonly shared among other workers. Understanding that other people *also* often feel physically stuck and unable to move while time slows to a crawl in the moment of not-knowing can both normalize and detraumatize this reaction when it recurs. Likewise, the realization that feelings of exposure and shame often arise during and after these moments can help youth workers debunk the perception that they alone are thought to be charlatans. Remembering that these reactions are normal and quite common affirms to the worker that although the event remains uncomfortable and possibly embarrassing, using the theater metaphor described in chapter 7, one is not alone on the stage.

NOT-KNOWING CANNOT BE PREVENTED

Youth workers are often motivated by a desire to be helpful, to solve problems, and to alleviate suffering. It is not surprising, then, that one of the most common reactions to this study has been the immediate desire to learn how to prevent, interrupt, or explain moments of not-knowing. For instance, upon hearing the group home vignette in chapter 1 during a workshop, one worker immediately began problem-solving, suggesting that the youth worker in the story had simply misunderstood and inappropriately personalized the young woman's reaction. He went on to suggest that this reflects a training issue; if the worker had been properly trained to recognize and understand common reactions to trauma, the client's reaction would not have created such a moment of stuckness. Therefore, he added, not-knowing is a feature of poor preparation, a lack of training, and as such it can be prevented by adequately training youth workers for any and all scenarios.

What this worker missed was the recognition that experiences of stuckness are what they are not because of the details of the event but because of each individual worker's embodied response, in the moment, to that moment. They cannot be rationally explained away and dismissed, because they are not purely cognitive experiences. Nor do they result solely from a lack of education or perspective. They simply occur. Although they may occur to workers who are new to the field—where lack of training or experience may perhaps be a factor—moments of not-knowing also strike youth workers with advanced degrees and decades of experience. Since there is no way to anticipate or predict the confluence of events and circumstances that might constitute stuckness for any given worker on any given day, it is unrealistic to assume that not-knowing *can* be prevented.

It is not enough to say that not-knowing cannot be avoided. In fact, youth workers do themselves a disservice by believing that it *should* be. Stuckness and moments of not-knowing are features of youth work, and both workers and their clients are better served by understanding and working within these moments than focusing their attention on avoiding them. Indeed, as workers like Athena and Martin suggested when they discussed the power of winging it in chapter 9, developing the ability and willingness to recognize and sit with their own moments of stuckness allows youth workers a unique opportunity to engage with their clients, sharing the uncertainty and anxiety that comes with exploring unfamiliar terrain together. In this way, preventing not-knowing can be seen as limiting the range of experiences youth workers and clients share and from which they can learn. Recognizing that not-knowing is common and normal in the helping relationship allows youth workers to carry themselves with greater openness and accessibility to the young people they serve.

BLAME THE MYTH OF SUPERCOMPETENCE, NOT NOT-KNOWING

The desire to prevent, eliminate, or "solve" youth workers' stuckness is seductive; it is easy to become invested in the quest to prevent something that causes such discomfort. That same desire, however, deflects the attention away from the real problem illustrated by youth workers' descriptions of not-knowing. Seldom are the details of the events in which they became stuck responsible for the shame, vocational anxiety, and professional burnout described by the participants in this study. Not-knowing itself is not the problem. Instead, the problem rests in youth workers' reactions to the moment, which occur in a professional context that continues to reinforce the notion that not-knowing indicates incompetence and personal failure. The pain of not-knowing comes fundamentally from the myth of supercompetence and the degree to which youth workers believe in it.

After all, encountering a situation one does not know how to manage outside the professional context is commonplace; family members routinely stump one another with strange behaviors or expectations, travelers are often left despondent and uncertain in the face of a cancelled flight, and students regularly struggle to muddle through assignments they do not immediately understand. What differentiates these mundane experiences of not-knowing from those encountered in professional life is the perception that, as professionals, youth workers *must not* be in a situation where they are unable to respond. It is the commitment to Brown's (1980) moral component of the profession; ours is the responsibility to help. That, coupled with the profession's code of silence prohibiting colleagues from sharing moments in which they too were stuck, creates the trauma and anxiety of not-knowing: I do not know what to do, but as a professional I *should*, and anyone else in my shoes *would*, so what does this say about me? The narratives in this study reinforce that the problem is not not-knowing—that is merely a normal and healthy result of fallible human beings trying to be helpful—but rather the belief that in order to be helpful, we must be infallible.

ATTENDING TO EXPERIENCE IS POWERFUL

As the narratives in this study demonstrate, there is considerable benefit to be discovered by attending to how people experience events, not merely what they do or why they do it. Certainly, the latter questions are important for supervisory and practical reasons; it is essential to know what circumstances led to an event, what actions a youth worker took to resolve the situation, and why those actions were selected. However, workers in this study mentioned time and time again that as long as the discussions about their moments of stuckness focused solely (or even primarily) on these technical questions, they remained confused, anxious, and alienated as a result of their own reactions to these moments.

Phenomenological interviewing, even in its most rudimentary form, allows workers to explore with one another and in supervision not only what they did, what struggles they encountered in their work, but also how they experienced and made meaning of those struggles. This is not to say that the study suggests that all youth workers ought to become phenomenological researchers. Rather, phenomenology—attending directly to lived experience and meaning-making of events—is a useful orientation for practice and collegial consultation. In fact, personalizing and reflecting in this way on the experience, using questions designed to elicit descriptions of lived body, lived time, lived space, and lived relationship, can be an intervention in its own right for workers and clients alike. It can encourage workers to reflect in a new way on experiences and their reactions to them and open additional insight in the process. This style of interviewing—of conversation—invites deep reflection and connection between event and experiencer in a way that mirrors the introspection youth workers ask of their clients.

NOW WHAT? TRANSLATION TO PRACTICE

Having interviewed 12 youth workers for this study and discussed its findings with many more helping professionals (youth workers, social workers, educators, hospice workers, grief counselors, and more) in workshops and presentations, I routinely come back to the question, "Now what?" What does the profession do with the insights these workers' stories offer? Overall, investigation into the experience of not-knowing clarifies that as a field, much work remains to be done in order to operationalize the lessons learned from these interviews. Although many of the action steps, both practical and theoretical, suggested by this study seem straightforward or simple, they are nevertheless essential to pushing the field forward in confronting the myth of supercompetence and helping youth workers—individually and collectively—recognize, learn from, and move through their moments of stuckness without being shamed or punished by them. The action plan that evolved from this study includes specific tasks for youth workers on the front lines, supervisors, and the profession as a whole.

APPLICATIONS FOR THE FRONT LINES

Individual front-line youth workers, those who have the most direct and doubtless most emotionally and often physically taxing interactions with young people, also have the most direct involvement and experience with moments of stuckness. Not surprisingly, not-knowing takes its most significant toll among these workers, and two of this study's practical applications are most relevant for them:

- Youth workers can use an increased awareness and understanding of not-knowing to recognize its features when they encounter them and grant themselves permission for the experience.
- Youth workers must develop collegial support networks in which these moments are discussed within a climate of safety and support, with the intent of breaking down a culture of silence that allows the myth of supercompetence to thrive in professional contexts.

BECOME A FALL JUNKY

During a presentation on this study to fellow academics, I began discussing the practical implications and utility of the research. One of the attendees interrupted to ask me, completely out of the blue, if I rock climb. Taken aback and puzzled (I'm anything but a rock climber), I replied that I have never climbed. This colleague went on to suggest that, from his perspective, the most useful and direct application of this research was analogous to the experience—among rock climbers—of falling. In the attempt to scale sheer cliffs, falling is inevitable. Most climbers know this to be true, but only those who have fallen enough times, and with enough reflection on their own practice and experience of falling, learn to enjoy the fall.

Among these climbers, whom my colleague called "fall junkies," the fall becomes as much a feature of the climb as a successful ascent. It is ideal, of course, to make a successful climb without falling, but it is accepted as an inevitable part of the process that even the most skillful climbers will, on occasion, fall. The challenge for reflective climbers is to attend so deliberately to their craft that they recognize the indicators that a fall is imminent; they learn to identify how their bodies feel, how the rock sounds, and what happens to their ropes just before the fall. Then, when their grip at last slips and they fall, they recognize that the rest is beyond their control; they have fallen before and must simply trust to their skill in placing their pitons and ropes and allow themselves to fall until they are stopped.

My colleague added that, in reflecting on the fall, fall junkies talk about the blend of elation, fear, energy, and faith they experience. They attend fully to the experience *first* and then discuss where their footing may have gone wrong and what corrections may be made in subsequent attempts. I knew in that moment that he had made the connection I had long sought for language to articulate, using a metaphor that was both foreign to me and surprisingly apt to the circumstance. The most relevant application of this study to youth work practice is that youth workers must learn to become fall junkies.

Of course, youth workers enter into their relationships with youth, indeed into each interaction with youth, with deliberate attention to plotting the best possible course to whatever outcome has been identified. The youth worker–young person relationship is carefully constructed and nourished, such that young people walk through a process of "connection, discovery, and purpose" (Krueger, 1998, p. 3) that results in healthy, accomplished adulthood. The youth worker is primarily responsible for reading the cues that indicate the best means to this end. In the metaphor of the rock climber, youth workers carry a professional obligation, in each interaction and relationship, to select a course up the cliff and help young people set their guide ropes and climb.

Nevertheless, moments occur in which, for whatever reason, the course becomes unclear and the youth worker begins to slip. The stories in this study have illustrated some of the embodied reactions or indicators that often accompany the fall into stuckness; they are youth work's equivalent of a shaky handhold or sliding rock.

The challenge, for workers as for climbers, is to recognize these moments as they build, correct if possible along the way, but allow themselves to fall when they must. The fall itself is difficult and sometimes frightening, certainly, but it need not be condemning; by learning to recognize the features of not-knowing as they unfold, youth workers can develop trust that their ropes are securely fastened, their harnesses snug and safe, and accept that falling is, evidently, a feature of this particular climb. Better still, falling is not only a static feature, but in its entirety can be experienced as a moment of vocational potential.

Critical and meaningful reflection, of course, must follow the fall; without this reflection and introspection, the experience offers little in terms of instruction for subsequent experiences. As with the climber, the youth worker after moments of not-knowing stands much to gain from remembering, talking about, and reflecting on the meaning of each individual fall. This will not prevent falls in the future—that is, after all, not the goal—but it may help to contextualize that particular fall and open the possibility of new insight into how to set the ropes and select a course in the next attempt on that particular wall.

This is perhaps the most significant practical contribution of embracing the fall; in youth work, the moment of not-knowing can open possibilities with clients. Lesser (2005) and Ricks and Bellefeuille (2003) have suggested that in the helping relationship, *knowing* has the potential to blind professionals to unexplored possibilities in their practice, and that a deliberate stance of not-knowing may open these possibilities. Athena and Martin, two participants in this study, offered a similar perspective. The recognition of the fall, the moment of stuckness, can remind the youth worker that, as her clients often do not know where they are headed and often fall without warning, it personalizes and deepens the helping relationship for youth workers to walk a short mile in those shoes, as well. By learning to embrace the fall of not-knowing rather than punishing themselves for the incompetence they fear it reflects, youth workers position themselves to chart a new course *with* their clients, rather than merely on their behalf. They model that it is okay to fall, that the human experience is fallible, one of trial-and-error, and that the goal of the climb—while it may ultimately involve reaching the summit—is to live the adventure along the way.

CREATE NETWORKS OF SUPPORT

To push the climbing metaphor a little further before abandoning it, no accomplished climber climbs alone; the risk of injury is simply too great. Likewise, the risk of vocational, emotional, and psychic injury from the shame and silence associated with not-knowing is too great for youth workers to continue going it alone. Youth workers, in sharing their moments of stuckness with me, said time and time again that they never told these stories to their peers for fear of judgment and shame. Some, like Cleve, openly acknowledged that they had been reluctant even to share them with me, in the safety and anonymity of a research project. This climate of shame and fear speaks to the pervasive and condemning power of the myth of supercompetence and must be addressed.

A twofold response is necessary. On an individual level, youth workers must seek to understand their experiences of not-knowing in the context of others, becoming fall junkies. At the same time, workers must begin to develop opportunities where and when these experiences can be shared, interpreted, and internalized. Such collective actions have long been accepted as models of best practice for helping professionals working with trauma victims as attempts to manage and prevent vicarious traumatization (McCann & Pearlman, 1990), and residential staff in Arieli's (1997) study of discontent in residential child and youth care suggested that this reflective practice—including the sharing of experience with colleagues—may be effective in decreasing experiences of discontent. Nevertheless, professional versions of mutual-aid groups have yet to establish solid footing in many youth work environments.

These supportive networks, of course, need not be extraordinarily formal or organizationally rooted; they may emerge organically among colleagues in the form of monthly lunches dedicated to processing their reactions to their work (as distinct from more conventional case consultation, which often focuses on technical and practical dilemmas presented by clients' circumstances). The structural details of these networks notwithstanding, it is essential that they consist of youth work colleagues and ideal that these professional peers represent a diverse mix of experience and education, as it is the fear of judgment and inferiority that fuels the myth of supercompetence and entrenches not-knowing as an indicator of shame and incompetence.

APPLICATIONS FOR SUPERVISION

Youth workers on the front line, although most likely to encounter critical moments of stuckness, are not without allies in addressing, responding to, and learning from these experiences. Supervisors are well positioned to support their staff in interpreting and making meaning of these challenging professional dilemmas, helping them to become significant learning opportunities in an individual worker's professional development rather than sources of shame and vocational anxiety. Specifically, supervisors and administrators have the potential to structure their activities with staff such that they balance technical details, attention to practical problem-solving, and workers' personal, lived experiences and reactions to the very problems for which supervision is necessary.

Unfortunately, constraints of time and resource often force supervisors to focus the majority of their attention on the technical and practical elements of their staffs' work, as illustrated in the group home vignette described in chapter 1. In their narratives of stuckness, youth workers admitted that the supervision immediately following their experiences emphasized technical issues: What did you do? Why did you do it? What would you do similarly or differently in the future? Although the circumstances in which their not-knowing moments were addressed, their personal reactions to those moments were not. No participant in the study made this observation with any malice; in fact, all were quite complimentary of their supervisors. Nevertheless, many left their supervision meetings feeling even more alienated and anxious about their reactions to not-knowing than they had before they entered. The unintended consequence of a primary supervisory emphasis on technical problem-solving is the reinforcement of a silence around the personal toll exacted by not-knowing.

Certainly, it goes without saying that attending to technical and practical problem-solving is a central feature of supervision; it is clearly needed to assure quality of services delivered to youth and essential to the ongoing professional development and skill-building of staff. Still, supervision must also include opportunities and explicit invitations for exploration of reflective and personal reactions to the stressful events so common in youth work. Anglin (2002) has written of the need for such ongoing supervision in order for residential workers to develop mindful and reflective practice. His study of residential care facilities suggested that well-functioning facilities are those in which care-work teams are adequately and supportively supervised.

Phenomenological technique offers a deliberate and sound method by which supervisors can facilitate thoughtful introspection and experiential meaning-making for their staff. By attending first to technical details of a given event, the supervisor and youth worker create a shared understanding of the circumstances giving rise to that event and process the practical lessons the experience may offer. Taking that shared framework and allowing it to stand as a scaffolding for the worker's experience of the events, supervisors can then move with their staff into explorations of the lived experience: What was the moment really *like* for the worker? Ehrich (2005) has suggested similar applications of phenomenological research methods in management, providing a framework for drawing out human experiences in that field. In youth work, eliciting such descriptions allows workers to be heard in fullness, without the perceived need to bracket their personal experiences from their professional consultation, and creates a climate in which authentic reflective practice (Palmer, 1998) may emerge.

APPLICATIONS FOR THE PROFESSION

Youth work in the United States is a profession in formation. Many, if not most, workers receive little or no formal training in youth work theory or practice, learning the majority of their skill through direct experience on the job. Youth workers remain underpaid and often undervalued, ever seeking the public's recognition of their authority to work with and on behalf of young people. The field strives to carve out its own well-articulated practical and theoretical space somewhere between its parent disciplines of social work and formal education, drawing from each but remaining distinct from both. In this climate, it is hardly surprising that youth workers hold themselves to the myth of supercompetence, an ideal of practice in which uncertainty or stuckness is perceived to be paramount to incompetence and therefore stigmatized.

However, youth workers operate in environments that are in constant states of change, often chaotic, and utterly unpredictable. No amount of training or experience can possibly equip a worker to respond immediately and effectively to every situation encountered in the course of a working relationship with young people. Nevertheless, functioning under an emerging conception of professionalism that stresses autonomous decision-making and the ability to respond systematically and effectively to situations encountered in professional activities, youth workers often associate their own experiences of not-knowing what to do as indications of incompetence that threaten professional identity.

What does this mean for the field and for the survival of the skilled, competent, and humanly fallible youth workers in it? This study of not-knowing has illustrated that the field must undergo a redefinition of professionalism as it is lived in youth work. Similar to the discipline of child care and early childhood education (Powell, 1990), youth work must redefine professional identity, retain an emphasis on developing codes of ethics as well as an established theory base and associated skill set, and value professional autonomy but challenge the false polarity that knowing indicates competence and not-knowing represents the opposite. As a profession, youth work must come to embrace the power and potential to be realized by admitting to its own fallibility while setting high standards for reflective practice and integrated supervision that allow workers to walk as partners with youth, charting a careful and deliberate course, setting the guide ropes responsibly, and embracing the fall as part of the adventure. By accepting that stuckness is as much a feature of effective, engaged, competent youth work as is goal attainment and achievement of treatment goals, youth work can lead the helping professions in debunking the myth of supercompetence and be nourished by authentic, reflective practice in the process.

PARTING THOUGHTS: IT'S LIKE TAXES

My favorite part of the interview process is the moment near the end, as the tape recorder winds down and the notes are being put away. Having spent an hour or two (or three) together, sharing some of the deepest emotional secrets of the profession, these are the moments when participants and I feel closest to one another. We understand one another better than at any other point in the process. We have developed a rapport, a sense of trust and shared interest. These are the times when the most honest, the deepest, and the most pure impressions of their work come through. These are the conversations most in need of sharing. They offer more to the field, to the understanding of not-knowing, than any number of pages of my reflections.

I remember this moment in my conversation with one worker, Martin. It was a hot summer day and we sat at his kitchen table, sipping from our glasses and relaxing for a moment. The tape recorder was still running as Martin reflected on his years of experience in the field. He has done youth work, in the same agency and virtually the same position, for nearly 20 years. Using that history as a framework, Martin started telling me about the price he has seen youth workers pay for their failure to talk honestly with one another about their personal and professional struggles, of which the moment of not-knowing may be one of the most significant. We talked about burnout and alienation. He told me about what he perceived to be the stuckness of youth work culture, that we operate as though not-knowing is shameful and therefore pretend it doesn't exist. There were several times in the conversation when he lowered his eyes to the table and his voice got very quiet, as though he had withdrawn into himself.

After one of those moments, Martin looked at me and told me that we need to stop seeing not-knowing as only draining. We need to learn to see it as opportunity, at the same time. Of course, it's uncomfortable. Of course, we don't like it. But remembering that it exists is part of what keeps us accessible to the youth we serve. Being cast off the mythical throne of omnipotence is the healthiest thing we can do, he said. At the same time, it is threatening, but only as long as we try to hide it from our peers or our supervisors. Martin stressed that the more we learn to be attentive to what it is like for us to experience not-knowing (what it feels like, what it means for us later on, and what it means for our clients), the more complete and human we can be for the youth we serve. By sharing these moments, we can embrace existential humility, debunk the myth of supercompetence, and see ourselves more truly. The payoff, he said, "is in debriefing with similar workers, and [using that moment to] understand our own process . . . our internal process . . . [and to understand] ourselves better. That feels really enriching."

I remember asking how to reconcile what is enriching about reflecting on the moment of not-knowing with what is difficult and painful about living through it. Although his was only my second or third interview, in that moment, Martin shared with me an image that I knew would be the conclusion to this study. He said that not-knowing is like taxes. No one likes to pay them. They sometimes cause significant distress in the short-term. If unattended, they can cause huge problems for us down the road. But, he said, "Taxes are enriching. Taxes aren't something that just gets taken away. They then feed us back in other ways. They pay for things. And that's exactly the right word. [Not-knowing] is taxing."

REFERENCES

Anglin, J. (2002). *Pain, normality, and the struggle for congruence: Reinterpreting residential care for children and youth.* New York: The Haworth Press.

Arieli, M. (1997). *The occupational experience of residential child and youth care workers: Caring and its discontents.* New York: The Haworth Press.

Brown, M. M. (1980). *What is home economics education*? Minneapolis, MN: Minnesota Research and Development Center for Vocational Education, Department of Vocational and Technical Education, University of Minnesota.

Ehrich, L. (2005). Revisiting phenomenology: Its potential for management research. In *Proceedings: Challenges for organizations in global markets* (pp. 1–13). British Academy of Management Conference, Said Business School, Oxford University.

Krueger, M. (1998). *Interactive youth work practice.* Washington, DC: CWLA Press.

Lesser, Y. (2005). Potential space: Knowing and not knowing in the treatment of traumatized children and young people. *British Journal of Social Work, 37*, 23–37.

McCann, L., & Pearlman, L. A. (1990). Vicarious traumatization: A framework for understanding the psychological effects of working with victims. *Journal of Traumatic Stress, 3*, 131–149.

Palmer, P. (1998). *The courage to teach: Exploring the inner landscape of a teachers' life.* San Francisco: Jossey-Bass.

Powell, D. R. (1990). Professionalism and the child care field: What model? *Child & Youth Services, 13*(1), 177–186.

Ricks, F., & Bellefuille, G. (2003). Knowing: The critical error of ethics in family work. *Child and Youth Services, 25*, 117–130.

Appendix A: Interview Guide

APPENDIX A: INTERVIEW GUIDE

Not Knowing What to Do: A Study of Youth Workers, Stuckness, and the Myth of Supercompetence

Interviews will involve two stages. In the first interview, participants will be asked to describe a situation of not-knowing from their work. The second will be a follow-up interview to check for resonance of the tentative themes.

Interview I

- Think of a work situation during which you experienced "being stuck" or "not knowing what to do." Tell me about that situation:
  - Where did it take place?
  - How long did it last?
  - How long did it seem to last?
- Imagine yourself in that moment: What was it like to be you?
- What was your body doing? What was it like to be in your body?
- What was time doing in that situation? What was it like to be aware of time?
- What meanings did you make from this experience? What meaning do you make from it now?

Follow-Up Interview

- What did you notice about my interpretation?
- How did my interpretation of your story fit (or not) with your experience of you in it?
- Are there places where my reading and your reading are the same? Different?

- Should I change things about my interpretation of your story? What should I change?

Additional Prompts

- I'm interested by what you just said. Can you tell me more about what you mean by "_______?"
- That's a phrase I haven't heard you use yet. Can you tell me what that means?
- I want to make sure I understand you right. Do you mean _______?

Index